Beyond the Next Village

Beyond the Next Village

A Year of Magic and Medicine in Nepal

Mary Anne Mercer

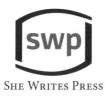

SHE WRITES PRESS

Published 2022
Printed in the United States of America
Print ISBN: 978-1-64742-343-8
E-ISBN: 978-1-64742-344-5
Library of Congress Control Number: 2021923639

For information, address:
She Writes Press
1569 Solano Ave #546
Berkeley, CA 94707

She Writes Press is a division of SparkPoint Studio, LLC.

For Sita
my Nepali sister

and

for my mother

Somewhere children dance to the joyous music of life
and elsewhere they only cling to existence.
They are all ours.

—*Laurie Kohl*

Contents

Prologue
Nepal, 1978

I reached over to take the wrist of Maya, the young Nepali woman lying on a straw mat on the porch of her thatched-roof house. A crowd of family members and neighbors pressed in closely around us, all eyes focused on me.

Will she die? was the unasked question.

I was looking at a very sick woman, already in shock. Her pulse was weak and very rapid, a faint tapping against my fingers. Her face had a ghostlike sheen. I reached under her cummerbund to feel her abdomen and found it rigid, board-like. She groaned, opened her eyes briefly with a faintly pleading look, and closed them again.

I murmured softly, *"Pet dukhyo, hoina?" Your stomach hurts, doesn't it?* She moved her head faintly in response.

Maya's husband had confirmed that she was a few weeks pregnant. I tried to imagine a scenario that would end well for this woman and her worried husband, but all that emerged was fear that she would die unless she had surgery very soon.

I had been in rural Nepal for six months, leading a health team trekking village to village to provide immunizations and a few other health services. By default, I offered simple health care when people came to me with their everyday aches and pains. As a nurse practitioner in the US, I had learned diagnosis and treatment of common illnesses, and I knew which patients needed referral to more specialized medical services.

But the rules from home didn't seem to apply here. With no other help available, I found I had no choice but to do whatever was needed—even though that often meant overreaching my training.

We were in Gorkha, at a time when the entire district had no internal roads at all. The only way to get Maya surgical care was a mission hospital, ten hours' walk away, via rocky footpaths. It was adequately staffed and equipped, but if the doctor happened to be gone, the trip would be for naught. And was there time to get her there before she succumbed?

"She's very sick," I said quietly to the husband after finishing a cursory exam. He gave a sideways Nepali nod, with a look of grim concern.

"*Ke garne?*" he muttered, as if reluctant to hear the answer. *What to do?*

My clinical mind went back and forth, weighing choices, balancing fear for Maya and reasonable possibilities for action. Was there even a best option? If she stayed home, she would have the care and comfort of her those who loved her, in her own culture, but with only a small chance she would survive. How to balance those odds? Finally, I advised her husband that if she could be taken to the mission hospital on a stretcher, it might be possible for her to have an operation that would save her life. He looked back at me blankly, either not understanding or not believing my words. But after consulting with several other men on the scene, and finding some to help, he agreed.

After several false starts and delays, Maya was moved onto a stretcher improvised from a heavy blanket suspended between two poles. As the four men carrying her passed out of sight down the trail, I was filled with questions that would haunt me my whole time in Nepal. Had I done the right thing? Would Maya survive the trip? I'd never before had the dilemma of making this kind of decision, weighing odds that had so little basis in medicine and so much to do with the poverty and injustice that was everyday life for rural Nepalis. What was my role here, in this world that was so unlike any I'd ever known?

Chapter 1
Arrival

What on earth have I done? I wondered, peering through the plane's window at my future, a few thousand feet below. Snow-laden craggy peaks stretched to the end of the visible world. I knew this was a pivotal moment. Was I ready to change my life?

The stupendous display of the Himalayan range was beautiful, but the mountains were cold, distant, frightening in their vastness. Both my hands gripped the seat arm nearest the window. I wanted to feel excited, elated, but an undercurrent of panic coursed through my body, threatening to burst out through my skin. I took a series of slow, deep breaths and willed myself to be calm, to enjoy this unique moment. This was my new life.

As we circled lower, I scanned the Kathmandu airport, looking for the fabled cattle on the runway that would make our landing a dangerous game of chance. The ground moved closer and I could make out a few cows near the airstrip, but none obstructing our path. Maybe just another international travelers' folktale, I decided, as we thumped down on the bumpy tarmac.

Having just maneuvered through the Hong Kong and Bangkok airports en route, I was prepared for the chaos of managing luggage, customs, and the visa inspection. But the Kathmandu airport was another step up in confusion and disorientation—total chaos! The directional signs all seemed misplaced, with doors blocked off and long lines formed for no discernible purpose. Eventually, I located my bags and passed all the required checkpoints.

As I emerged from the safety of the building, a mass of humanity surged forward to greet me. "Madam! I have cheapest taxi! Come this way," shouted dozens of frantic-looking men as they pushed each other aside, trying to grab my luggage. Horns blared, and the hungry roar of motorcycles added to the din. The stench of exhaust, unwashed bodies, and a vaguely moldy scent filled the steamy air. I clutched my bags closely, searching for the officially designated cabs I had been instructed to use.

Suddenly I had a foreboding image of what life in Nepal would be: alone, with endless stress and tension, confusion, and aggressive strangers wanting something from me. I felt myself cower inwardly, wanting to escape back to a place of comfort, of familiarity. But that was not an option.

Finally, I spied the signs for an "official" taxi and struggled through the crowd to reach one. The driver, standing by his door, looked at me impassively, slung my luggage into the trunk, and ushered me into the back seat. He gave a sideways nod of his head when I provided what I thought was a vague address, a house in a neighborhood of Kathmandu called Chabahil, and we set off—down the road to the past and the future all at once.

I had anticipated this day for most of my life, beginning with my first glimpse of the enchantment of other lands. Once, from the dusty country road of my Montana childhood, a strange car drove up the lane into our farmyard. The only traveling salesman we had ever seen was the Fuller Brush man, and this visitor was an astounding surprise, bringing not brushes but pure magic. He was from somewhere in the Middle East, small, swarthy, and very polite. After his first visit, he arrived every year to spread his treasures on our farmhouse kitchen table. The tapestries he sold were mysterious, woven with vaguely biblical-looking pictures on olive-toned satin, edged with shiny gold fringes. My mother, thirsty for all things foreign, would buy a few dresser scarves and other pieces of undetermined use. For a decade or more, they gathered dust on our end tables and the kitchen buffet, regular reminders that there was another world out there. Waiting.

I grew up on a ranch in the shelter of cottonwoods with rolling hills of short-grass prairie dominating the landscape. My large family and our dozen or so neighbors with solid roots in the land were my whole world. Travel to the nearest town was the only adventure most people seemed to need, but I always craved seeing a bigger world. By the time I left high school, my plan was to go to Asia after college to live out a dream of being in a totally different place on this earth. I would work as a nurse and learn about people who were nothing like anyone I had known. Was it the movies that spurred my interest in foreign settings? Ingrid Bergman serving orphans in China, or Mitzi Gaynor as a Navy nurse in the South Pacific? Or maybe my mother's intense fascination with the historic ruins of Europe, which she studied from an ancient set of maroon-bound books called *Stoddard's Lectures*. Like my mother, I wanted more, and I knew it was inevitable that I would leave Montana to see what else was out there for me.

I didn't journey to those foreign places for many years. Leaving our one-room country school for high school in town and then college was a frightening foray onto a stage where I struggled to fit in, learn small talk, wear the right clothes, and wonder who else I could be. Then, in college, I fell deeply in love with Bill, a charismatic dreamer, and succumbed to his insistence that we be together, marry, share our lives. We lived in San Francisco, Boston, Denver, Spokane, and again in San Francisco. The marriage lasted eight years, and all the while I left my dream tucked away in a box marked "someday."

Leaving this deeply flawed man was drawn out and intensely painful. We separated, reunited, separated again. Once the divorce was final, I was in a gray cave, fearing that a patch of daylight would never appear. I despaired of finding my way out.

After months of darkness, one morning I opened a greeting card from my mother showing a bright yellow sunrise and the well-known maxim: "Today is the first day of the rest of your life." Finally, it was.

I enrolled in nurse practitioner training just down the street from my Sunset District flat in San Francisco. After finishing the program, a position as the director of a charming community clinic in the North Beach/Chinatown area dropped into my lap. Suddenly, I was living the single life to the fullest, with a great job and a wide array of friends, men and women, straight and gay, Americans and internationals, doctors, lawyers, and college dropouts. I was mysteriously "popular" in a way that I had never been in my earlier life as student and then wife. I fell into relationships with men easily, quickly, always surprised at their interest and availability. My friends laughed, calling me the "gay divorcée," an archetype from a 1930s movie of that name. I was out every night, rarely alone. Though I knew I was running from the pain and loneliness of having split with my husband, I could imagine no alternative to this frantic busyness.

Then a college friend, Margaret, came to visit. She was a world traveler, an artist, a student of cultures. She had just returned from Nepal and could talk of little else. We sat in a small café one evening, and she told me about the wonders of Kathmandu.

"It's the most fascinating place I've ever been," she told me. "If there was only one country you should see before you die, it would be Nepal. It's unique, a world apart."

Not long after Margaret left, I was randomly scanning the Sunday paper want ads and saw in bold type: "NURSES WANTED, NEPAL." I was stunned. Nurses. Nepal. Wanted now. I realized at that moment that the "someday" I dreamed of had just materialized.

The following week, I took a break from my clinic, hopped on a cable car to the address listed in the ad, and interviewed with the kindly older woman who had placed it. She represented a nonprofit foundation that had a long history of health efforts in Nepal. The position was for a volunteer and paid only a small stipend plus all expenses. I would sign up for eighteen months to work with another American nurse conducting an immunization campaign in a rural area.

Even before finishing the interview, I knew that I would take the position, leave my life in San Francisco, and jump into that future that I had wanted for so long. Three weeks later, I was on a plane to Nepal.

The taxi set out on a jerky, swerving ride down a narrow dirt road-way from the Kathmandu airport to my new residence. The street was lined with red mud-brick houses with thatched or tile roofs that looked as though they could be centuries old. In the space of five minutes, I had a sudden flash of wonder: I'd come to live in not just another country, another continent, but another time altogether. I was overwhelmed with the fuzzy, this-makes-no-sense feeling of being in a dream—or drugged—in some unknown medieval setting. It was real, but in the same way that dreams or movies seem real but are immaterial, imaginary.

Before long the street was filled with people of all ages, the men and children in Western clothes, the women dressed in long wrap-around skirts in various faded dark patterns. They were on foot, on bicycles, carrying loads, carrying toddlers, herding goats, and step-ping around chickens and cows that seemed to have full right-of-way. Very young children, in ragged clothes with unwashed faces, played together with no adults in view. The harsh late morning sun shone on piles of trash lining the road, and the rank smell of rotting garbage wafted in the taxi window at regular intervals.

No matter who or what was in the direct path of our vehicle, the driver sped on at a steady pace, and people and animals drifted out of our path apparently without noticing us. My initial panic at thinking we were about to smash headlong into a passing cow turned to admiration for the driver's skills in maneuvering through the chaotic human and animal traffic. Passing and meeting other vehicles was another part of the seamless choreography of that taxi ride. By the time we reached the office house, I was convinced that my taxi driver would be fully qualified to take on the Indy 500.

What came next was almost as surreal as traveling down a medieval roadway. We pulled up to an elegant white mansion surrounded by a high brick wall, with a guard looking out from an imposing set of wrought-iron gates. I could see beds of brilliantly colored flowers beyond the gate. The driver stepped out to speak to the guard, and it was quickly determined that this was the right place.

"Here, madam," said the driver, ushering me out of the cab. *Madam.* I suddenly was something of a personage, arriving at my palatial home, away from the rabble of the streets. I was safe now, but also oddly uneasy at the sight of this luxury in contrast to the scenes I had just traveled through.

The Foundation's country director greeted me when I arrived at the house. Greta was a cool, slim woman in a primly tailored cotton dress, who spoke with a German accent. "You must be Mary Anne. Please come in. How was your trip?" Without waiting for an answer, she went on, "You're exhausted, I'm sure. Let's have some tea. Maya, *chia leraao,*" she beckoned to a smiling young woman standing by the door.

"Thank you so much—something to drink would be perfect. I really am quite tired," I murmured, sinking into an easy chair. Maya soon brought a tray with an elegant china tea service and plates of cookies. My mind was a mess of fatigue, confusion, curiosity, jet lag, and exhilaration, so I was happy to sit quietly and sip the strong milky concoction.

Greta asked courteously again about my travels and then launched into a briefing about some problems in the health team that I would be joining after my language training. Having had very little prior orientation about the specifics of the field activity, I listened mutely, trying to appear as if I understood. In fact, I had been given scant information about the job I had come to do, other than the basic facts. As this wasn't the right time to find out more, I sat quietly while she chattered on. She assured me that I could come to her for any questions or problems I might encounter and quickly took her leave.

I immediately climbed the elegant staircase to my bedroom, where my luggage had been delivered. Without any attempt at unpacking, I dropped onto the brocade bedspread, relishing the soft foam comfort in the cool, quiet room. Blessed relief from the stresses of the day enveloped me, and I drifted off into an exhausted slumber.

When I woke it was nearly dark. I could make out the faint glow of a reddish sunset shining through the windows and the outline of furniture here and there. For a moment, I wondered where I was. It came in a flash. *I'm here, I'm in Nepal. What now?* Hearing voices downstairs, I sat up, ran my fingers through my hair, and ventured out.

Following the sounds downstairs to the dining room, I was greeted by two smiling young women seated at the large mahogany table. They introduced themselves as Margie, an American, and Genevieve, who was French. They were fellow volunteers, videographers who had come to make a film of the activities of the Foundation.

"So you've met Greta," noted Margie. She was boyishly dressed, with short black hair. "Let me introduce you to the house staff." She led me around to meet the two Nepali staff members still in the house: Maya, the pretty young woman who had served the tea, was the maid, and Prem was the cook, a small wiry older man who was apparently busy preparing the evening meal. They each smiled deeply and gave me a namaste greeting: head slightly bowed, hands folded as if in prayer. I'd read that, roughly translated, namaste meant "I honor the light within you."

Maya and Prem were more prosperous-looking versions of the people I had passed on the road. I wondered what it was like for them to work in these luxurious surroundings, and then to go home to that other world outside.

"We also have a gardener, Gambir, and some guards, but I don't know their names," added Genevieve in her lilting French accent. "And drivers and a *dhobi,* who does the laundry. You'll get used to being waited on here. It's not so bad," she said with a smile.

Margie showed me around the house, which was indeed palatial. The first level floors were marble, and the five huge bedrooms upstairs had elegant parquet flooring and built-in mahogany closets. A tiled deck graced the roof. She pointed out the commanding view from my bedroom: Kathmandu valley, the mountains, and Bodnath, a famous Buddhist stupa nearby.

"You must be hungry," Margie commented when we had finished the tour. "We waited to eat so we could all have dinner together."

In the dining room we sat down at the large formal table to a meal of curried chicken, rice, and a type of squash I didn't recognize. I was suddenly ravenous and dug in appreciatively. When I asked for seconds, Prem, who was standing by, gave a pleased smile.

"*Meetoh?*" he asked. I looked at him blankly, wondering what to say.

"That means delicious," commented Genevieve.

"Oh yes, very *meetoh!*" I replied enthusiastically, and he smiled again as he retired to the kitchen.

The three of us chatted about where we had each come from, our lives before Nepal. Margie began to tell me what I might expect of the next few weeks, with warnings about culture shock.

"Don't be surprised if absolutely everything is strange for a while," she said sympathetically. "There is so much that's new, it'll be hard to take it all in. And having some familiar reminders of home will be important, such as books or music. Did you bring any of that?"

I listed some of the cassette tapes I'd thrown into my duffle bag at the last minute—John Denver, The Beatles, Carly Simon—and Margie nodded approvingly.

What I didn't mention was the internal struggle I had gone through as to what music to bring with me and what to leave behind. So many of the '70s songs spoke to me about the end of my marriage, the pain of looking back onto something I had loved and lost: Joan Baez's "Diamonds and Rust," the yearning to be Anne Murray's "Snowbird" and fly away from betrayal. I hadn't wanted to bring all that pain with me but realized at some level that I was leaving behind much more than music. So I had brought a bit of everything: rock, folk, and some orchestral classics. Those cassettes stayed with me as I explored some decidedly unfamiliar places over the next year.

A fixed daily routine began just two days later. After being served breakfast (of my choice, with linen napkins on gold-rimmed china), I went by bicycle to Nepali language classes. Returning to the house at five, exhausted after six intensive hours of one-on-one instruction, I was served dinner with the other women and then retired to the quiet privacy of my room.

I soon learned that having house staff meant I was taken care of totally—they shopped, cooked, cleaned, did the laundry, even made my bed in the morning. I had a driver at my disposal if needed. *Ah, this is why people want to be wealthy!* I thought. Initially, I felt grateful that I would be looked after in this foreign environment, where I hadn't the faintest idea how I would cope on my own. I'd later see that having a lavish lifestyle that would be unaffordable in their home countries was a key element of many expatriates' decision to work internationally.

Yet the idea of having servants also made me uneasy. I was used to having ranch help in my childhood; our "hired man" lived as one of the family, taking his meals with us and sharing holidays and special events. The rural setting of my upbringing was so nonhierarchical that seeing the privilege that came with my simply being foreign here was already a niggling discomfort.

Those first few days were a jumble of new people, reactions, and sensations as I tried to orient myself to an entirely new environment. I was overwhelmed by the massive inputs of sights, sounds, smells, and feelings, struggling to put them in some sort of order. This was not just another country; it was a wholly different civilization. My forays on the bicycle during the day solidified my growing sense of time warp about life in Kathmandu that I had felt on arrival. I carried my new Pentax camera, acquired during a layover in Hong Kong, with me everywhere. I wanted to photograph everything I saw, yet I ended up taking very few pictures, overwhelmed with all the possibilities. Even without photos, the images of the faces and the life in the streets stayed with me for many years.

The geography of Kathmandu itself was intriguing. The streets were laid out randomly, in nothing resembling squared-off grid lines. Some streets were paved but with huge potholes, others cobbled, many just wide dirt paths. The street names weren't marked. In fact, most seemed not to be named at all, referred to only by the neighborhoods they transected: Tangal, Dili Bazaar, Thamel. Many of the dusty orange-red brick houses were dilapidated and ancient-looking, but in some neighborhoods they had elegant carved wooden balustrades, windows, and door frames. Some fronted very closely against the street, others were set back into unkempt courtyards. Trash of all kinds was generously strewn about, including food remnants coated with flies and cow dung. A cacophony of sounds from the motors and horns of passing buses and cars was constant. Look-alike short-haired yellow dogs, skinny and sniffing through the trash for food, seemed to live in every neighborhood. *They all look like Scotty!* I thought with a pang of homesickness, one of our longest-lived childhood pets.

Pedaling down the streets, I caught glimpses of lives I'd never imagined. People walked or cycled down the center of the roadways and seemed mildly surprised when annoyed motorists honked to get past them. Pale beige cows, which I knew were sacred among this predominantly Hindu population, ambled freely, even in and out of the housing compounds. Chickens and goats abounded, along with naked babies in serious need of a good scrub. Most beautiful were the people: nearly all with shiny black hair but distinctive features. Some could have been olive-skinned Caucasians, others more clearly Asian or perhaps Middle Eastern. Nearly all were small in stature, with marvelous faces that could be impassively stony, then break into beautiful open smiles. They gave me friendly looks as I whirled by on my bicycle, some watching curiously. Their well-worn clothing spoke of poverty; only the school children looked washed and tidy, with white shirts, deep blue skirts or trousers, and book bags.

Every day something new on the ride would catch my eye. I wanted to take in everything I was seeing, to witness even more, to fill my memory with these fascinating scenes until my capacity to be amazed was saturated. But every evening, after a full grueling day of language training, I found myself retreating to the solitude of my room, writing in my journal and reading, escaping into a safe, familiar world.

After dinner near the end of my second week, as the sun was setting, I decided to explore the neighborhood on foot. My housemates had gone out, and I had begun to feel restless after staying indoors every evening. My tourist map showed me that Pashupatinath Temple, a major religious site on the banks of the holy Bagmati River, was not far away. *Time to get another look at where I am*, I mused. *Surely I can do that much on my own.*

I went out to the gate, smiled at the guard as he unlocked it for me, and began walking down the small dirt road that ran alongside the house. Very quickly, leaving the clamor of the main streets, I found another face of the city, this one dark, mysterious, and silent. The dirt road soon narrowed to a footpath and began to follow a small river, which I deduced was the Bagmati. The few scattered homes along the path, the small groups of people strolling near me, and the looming trees all took on that special almost-evening softening of outlines and fading of details. What might have been squalor in bright daylight was transformed into picturesque possibility. There was a haze in the air, blending the near and far dimensions into a decorative collage. Rounding a curve, I caught sight of the moon coming from behind the clouds—round, full, and yellow. I felt an amazing sense of peace in the air, blending with the murmur of the river and the calls of crickets, children, and jungle birds.

Finally, in the dim light I could see the complex of ancient buildings that was Pashupatinath, spreading along the river. I could make out clusters of pagoda-style roofs resting on intricately carved wooden rafters. As I continued along the path, statues and small shrines appeared on each side, with mysterious carvings on the walls behind them. Tiny kiosks lit only by small oil lamps loomed suddenly, with merchants selling offerings for the gods. Almost at the temple gate, I was startled by a throng of monkeys running back and forth along roofs and walls, chattering among themselves.

The main temple was forbidden to non-Hindus, so I continued past the temple gates along the path. The structures had been built in the fifth century, though restored or renovated several times since then. Lord Pashupati, one of the names of Lord Shiva, is known in Hinduism as the destroyer (the other two gods in the Hindu holy trinity being Brahma, the creator, and Vishnu, the preserver). Together the three gods represent the eternal process of creation, destruction, and regeneration.

A wide series of steps led down to the Bagmati River from the temple on both sides, providing easy access for the pilgrims to bathe in the river. Like any holy water, it would cleanse their souls of lifetimes of sins, I imagined, or complement the cremation rite for family members. I passed the main temple buildings, the remains of fires flickering on raised platforms along the river, and I realized that they were the burning *ghats*, open crematoria. The bodies had been placed on huge piles of wood, ceremoniously lit, and reduced to ashes. Placement at the edge of the Bagmati was strategic, so the ashes could be pushed into the river and flow eventually into the even holier Ganges, where every devout Hindu wants his or her ashes to be carried. It seemed fitting that the god who was known as the destroyer and transformer would preside over this site, where the earthly form of so many believers had ended.

I stood quietly for a while, stunned by the enormity of what I was seeing: the centuries of history that had passed through this place, the millions of devout Hindus who had connected with their gods here, the countless families who had bade farewell to their loved ones on these banks. The dimly lit scene seemed to me more a dream than the real world, or perhaps a waking hallucination. Finally, reluctantly, I turned to go.

A small but steady flow of travelers was leaving the temple, proceeding back in the direction I had come from. I joined them in the near darkness, making my way slowly back to my new, temporary home. Walking with them, wordless and filled with reverence and a new sense of peace, I felt that I was finally in Nepal. I was ready to live in this amazing civilization, to learn what it had to teach me. I had arrived.

Chapter 2

Sounding It Out

Each morning in language training, Jitendra and I sat facing each other on simple wooden chairs in a small room, with a blackboard on the wall and a rickety table by the door the only other furniture. Traffic noises from the street intruded through the open window, but closing it was not an option. It was sweltering, and there was no fan to provide any hint of a breeze.

Here I am, a kid again, I thought, struggling to focus, stay alert, and please my teacher. He looked at me with an encouraging and sympathetic smile.

"*Ma Nepali manche huu*," he enunciated slowly, as if saying to a child that he was a Nepali man.

"*Tapaai?*" You? With his longish hair slicked into place with some kind of pomade and his sparklingly white pressed shirt and black slacks, he reminded me of the Mormon missionaries who used to come to the door back home in Montana. He was just as pleasant, just as determined.

"*Ma Americaani aaimaai huu*." I answered back that I was an American woman, dreading the next step.

"*Raamro! Leknuos na*," was his reply—*Good, now write it.*

I groaned. Writing Nepali, more than just learning to speak the words, reduced me to the status of a frustrated six-year-old in her first week of school. I had always been a good student; I'd left San

Francisco just weeks before as a well-educated and respected health professional. Here, in a few short days I'd been reduced to an inarticulate child, struggling for hours at a time to remember simple words and phrases. It was beyond humiliating, a disturbing gap in my capabilities that I had never recognized before. I was good at French in high school. Why was this so hard? Would I ever be able to master the Sanskrit characters and recognize words without sounding them out?

Though my mom would be proud, I thought. As a teacher of remedial reading to grade schoolers, she was a champion of phonics, "sounding it out." My pitiful efforts to discover words behind the blur of similar-looking characters gave me great sympathy for that beginner's process of learning to turn lines on paper into recognizable sounds.

Spending six hours a day learning a wholly new language was excruciating. Though classified as an Indo-European language, it was very different from English, French, or Spanish, the languages I knew. With few of the same roots, every word had to be memorized without reference to familiar sounds. The sentence structure was at least mercifully simple, although also different from English. *He goes to town* became *he town to goes.*

On a typical morning I was exhausted and pleading for a break within an hour.

"*Guru-ji, ma ekdum taakaai laagyo,*" I pleaded my fatigue to Jitendra, feeling that my brain was about to congeal into a bowl of thick alphabet soup with Sanskrit characters milling about in constant random motion. "*Arum gaarnu paarcha.*" I needed to rest but hated my wheedling tone, pushing me further into child mode. *I'll bet I'm the worst student he's ever had!* I thought wistfully.

But Jitendra smiled patiently. "OK, shall we take a walk and talk about what we see on the street?" he asked.

"*Hunchha!*" I agreed, jumping up from my chair. We went out for a pleasant half hour of picking our way through the litter along the sides of the street and identifying objects around us. I tried to concentrate on remembering the words for what we passed as we walked: child, dog, chicken, house, cow, water, door, road. Mischievous-looking kids, who I estimated to be of school age but clearly weren't in school, watched us intently: the well-dressed Nepali man with the tall, pale-skinned, and light-haired foreign woman. We ambled along an open sewer here and there, but thinking it might be rude, I didn't comment on overwhelmingly rank smells that accosted us. Would he even notice it, I wondered, after living with these city odors all his life?

In the afternoons, my language teacher was Shambu. While Jitendra was tall, slim, and reserved, Shambu was shorter, muscular-looking, and very outgoing. He wore blue jeans and casual cotton shirts. The two young men also taught Nepali to Peace Corps volunteers, and both seemed to connect with what I was going through. They spoke casually about information related to the culture that I should know. The list of dos and don'ts gave me a growing awareness of the mysterious rules of this society I was entering. Rules such as: It's rude to point your feet at other people; feet are considered very unclean. The head is felt to be sacred, so never touch someone else's head. Use only the right hand for eating.

In contrast with serious Jitendra, Shambu was a jokey, hip young guy who worked at entertaining me as a part of his teaching. He recounted stories about Nepali history and fantastic tales from the Hindu religion, with its dozens and dozens of gods, each with a particular story.

"So what does it mean?" I asked on more than one occasion, trying to ferret out the deeper intention of what seemed to be folktales. "Is there a lesson behind it?"

"Oh, sometimes," he would reply. "Mostly it's just a story, something that was supposed to have happened a long time ago. We hear them when we're kids, but nobody explains them, really."

I could see, though, that Shambu's tales meant more to Nepalis than just the fanciful plots and characters; they were linked to childhood memories and shared events that I would never have access to. Similar to Santa Claus at Christmas and the roving bunny at Easter, no less fantastic, and just as hard to explain.

While language classes were exhausting, evenings and weekends offered relaxation. One night, my housemate Margie invited a British woman who was a Buddhist nun for dinner. A soft-spoken, articulate woman, Karen had closely cropped, curly blonde hair, a chunky silhouette, and wore dark red robes with various beads and amulets strung around her neck. I watched and listened with fascination as she related her story. She had a chronic illness that left her hardly able to walk that was, over time, cured by Tibetan medicine.

"It must have been amazing to finally recover from something so devastating," I commented after her story. "What did they find was the main problem? How were you treated?" I asked, feeling skeptical but wanting to hear more about this foreign medical miracle.

"The Tibetan doctors took months to find the root of the problem," she recounted. "They study many years to be able to identify the imbalances that make people sick. Treatments take a long time to work, too. I took herbs, did a lot of meditation. Finally my doctor made cuts in the skin on my back, and I got better."

"Wow, interesting," I mused, mentally running through the most likely biomedical diagnosis I could think of for her problems. A psychiatric problem called a conversion disorder, I thought, when neurological symptoms, such as blindness or paralysis, occur because of inner conflict after some very stressful experience. The Tibetan medicine could have helped her recover by convincing her that she would get better, not because of the treatments themselves.

But even with my skepticism about the efficacy of these strange-sounding practices (*cuts on her back?*), I had to wonder. Tibetan medicine was many centuries old. Did it make use of a type of knowledge that we didn't have? I couldn't have known then that I would soon encounter a range of ancient medical traditions over the next year, and how different those paradigms of healing would be from the kind of medicine I had studied and practiced. It was my first exposure to a whole new system of beliefs about causes and cures for illness.

One evening, Shambu invited me to his home for dinner with his family. I was elated—finally a chance to see inside a Nepali home, after so many days of riding past them on my bike. I hailed a cab on the main drag near the house, and showed the driver the directions Shambu had written down for me (actual addresses seemed rare in Kathmandu)—which of course I couldn't read, as they were jotted down in totally illegible Nepali script. We pulled up to a very simple frame building, in a complex of apartments.

I knocked, tentatively, on the main door, not certain it was the right place. Shambu opened it immediately and welcomed me in, smiling broadly, still in his blue jeans. Behind him was a lovely young woman in a dark-blue print sari, with two small children lurking behind her skirts. Pungent odors of frying garlic, onion, and spices filled the house, promising a memorable evening.

"Namaste, Mary Anne Didi. *Mero srimaati*, Barsha," he said, introducing me to his wife, who smiled shyly and gave a deep namaste. "Barsha doesn't speak much English," he said in a mildly apologetic tone. "And this is Bharat and Maya."

"*Namaste, and ekhdum dhaanyabaad* for having me over!" I smiled at the children and offered my thanks in an awkward mix of simple Nepali and English. "This is my first time in a Nepali home."

"You are most welcome," replied Shambu with a sweep of his hand inviting me to sit. "We are honored to have you. Our home is very simple, but I hope you enjoy the Nepali food." Barsha and the children immediately disappeared from the scene.

We sat down on a low-slung sofa with various snacks already set in front of us, and Barsha brought soft drinks with a smile and a nod. I gazed around the small room at the décor: pictures, mostly of Hindu gods or family members, hung high on the walls. Plastic flowers arranged in vases sat on a few pieces of dark wood furniture that seemed to reflect a more elegant past. The room was lit only by a single low-wattage bulb suspended from the high ceiling. We snacked and drank, snacked and drank for what seemed hours, chatting about his life, my life, what I was learning about Nepal.

Then my first authentic Nepali meal, different from the more Westernized food Prem served at the Chabahil house. It began with handwashing, using water poured from a pitcher over the hands and into a basin. Then Barsha brought in large shiny metal plates mounded with rice. Smaller metal bowls held the side dishes of lentils, curried vegetables, and nicely cooked liver, as well as a smaller dish of a tomato-onion-hot pepper mix. This basic meal was the ubiquitous Nepali staple I was to have twice daily for most of the year: dal (lentils) bhat (rice).

Shambu patiently showed me the traditional routine of eating without utensils. Step by step: First, with the (now clean) hands, move a little rice to one side of the plate, and with the fingertips mix a bit of the thin lentil mixture into the rice. Add some vegetables if desired. Then with the first three fingers, scoop up and spoon into the mouth a bit of the mixture, with the thumb following closely behind to guide it. If done correctly, a loud slurping sound should accompany the process.

The first time I tried it, some of the rice moved up into my palm, while most of the lentils dropped back onto the plate. "Whoops," I winced, looking up plaintively. "What did I do wrong?"

I was suddenly aware of the two small children standing in the doorway giggling uncontrollably. I grinned and made a funny face back at them. Shambu laughed too and said something with mock sternness to the children, who ducked out of sight.

"Ah, don't worry, just try it again," he responded. After a few more bites, I managed to get the food where it was supposed to go and began enjoying the rich flavors.

For the rest of the evening, Barsha came in regularly with more of everything and urged me to "eat more, eat more." Which I did, until I realized that the offers would continue to come until I was able convincingly to refuse. When we finished eating, I was able to exchange a few words with Barsha in a mix of English/Nepali, thanking her for the meal.

"Thank you so much for coming here," she said in her sweetly accented English, smiling. "Please to come again."

During the taxi ride home when the evening was over, I found myself reviewing the whole event. One image burned in my mind as the cab jostled along the rutted roadways: Barsha as the cook, but not as a participant in the meal. Why didn't she eat with us? I didn't ask Shambu, realizing that it must be the usual practice of Nepali families. But it was a question then, and for the entire rest of my time in Nepal: How do women live in this culture? How did it feel to be the family cook but be excluded from the meal with guests? Did she sense herself to be a servant as well as wife and mother of the household?

Learning to communicate in a new language included my first inkling of what it means to confront a different culture, including the frustrations of trying to understand it. Years later, my mantra when counseling young Americans who wanted to work overseas was: Spend time in that culture, long enough for it to begin to permeate your psyche—and not just intellectually. You need to actually be there, over time, to have even a small grasp of the meanings, the feelings that it evokes. Cultures can't just be "learned" as if they consist of simple information. Much later in my career I would encounter countless foreign aid projects that went astray because they were developed without the involvement of the people most affected, and with no real sense of local people's daily lives and deeply held beliefs.

✳

My first four weeks in Kathmandu passed by like a movie trailer, offering glimpses of an interesting story, but one I struggled to make sense of. The characters I met were fascinating, the setting was exotic, but as far as I could see there was no cohesive plot or meaningful action. Not yet. I kept watching, wondering how it would turn out.

During the second week of classes, I stopped at a popular Tibetan restaurant near the language school for lunch. The room was full of westerners, apparently tourists and trekkers given their backpacks and grubby appearance. Suddenly I was startled to see someone across the room who looked familiar. I struggled to identify the setting where this face belonged, and then light dawned: "Arnie!" I called, excited and incredulous. The man looked up, equally startled, and made his way across the room.

"Mary Anne! What on earth are you doing in Kathmandu?" he called out, sounding nearly as pleased as I felt. Arnie had been a pediatric resident at the hospital where I worked in San Francisco, a friendly guy with a great sense of humor whom we all liked immensely. He brought his lunch plate of Tibetan dumplings over to my table and we chatted excitedly, making plans to meet later.

The discovery that I knew someone from home gave a kind of lightness to my next few days. Arnie and his wife Olga seemed to also value meeting someone from home, and he was excited to show me their new little son, Simon. As the Peace Corps doctor and a US government employee, Arnie was happy to offer me access to the swimming pool, movies, and other events at the American Embassy compound. They introduced me to a few new restaurants that were mostly frequented by Americans and Brits, where we went occasionally for social events. It was comforting to spend time with people who looked like me, who knew the life I had left.

One evening I cycled across town to meet Arnie and Olga for

an American movie. I arrived with just a few minutes to spare, but Arnie had alerted the guard at the gate to the well-fortified embassy compound that I would be coming. Stashing my bike in the heavily guarded lot, I raced up to the simple frame building and spotted Arnie waiting for me.

"Arnie!" I called, breathless. "Sorry I'm almost late. Is Olga inside?"

Arnie smiled. "Nope, you're it for tonight. Simon had a fever, so she stayed home with him."

Going into the dimly lit hall, I did a momentary double take at seeing so few Nepalis and so many white faces, the most I'd seen in one place since I left San Francisco. Arnie and I made the rounds of the small crowd of casually dressed men and women, around my age or older, gathered outside the viewing room. Friendly, relaxed, they seemed to be mostly embassy or Peace Corps staff, with a few aid workers thrown in. The lights dimmed, and we went inside to find seats.

The plot of the movie was not particularly interesting, a comedy about kids and their dog rebelling against their parents. I laughed with the crowd, happy at being surrounded by people like me, part of a familiar activity. But as an everyday American urban scene appeared on the screen, I had an overwhelming surge of longing, a feeling of loss that blocked out everything else in the room. *Omigod, I think I might cry!* I thought. *Why?*

I closed my eyes and sucked all the air into my lungs that I could, blew it out, and pinched my mouth tightly closed. I realized how badly I wanted to see a well-kept yard with grass and familiar flowers, a clean street with curbs, a supermarket, an ice cream shop. Here there were no lawns, the streets were dirty, and there were no sidewalks worth the name. We were even advised not to eat ice cream because, made locally, it was not safe. I was homesick! The heaviness in my chest—the sense of loss, of loneliness—had been absent for a few days, but the silly movie brought it all back. Then the lights came on, and I was back in Kathmandu.

I cycled home in the dark, wondering how long it would take me to feel at home in this place that was such a contrast to the world I'd left. Restructuring my entire life had been a conscious choice, but as a result I was essentially stateless. Not a refugee seeking sanctuary from a war or a natural disaster like the millions forced from their homes every year—I couldn't imagine the misery they suffered. I had food, shelter, and work. No, this disquiet resulted from my own privilege, my good fortune. But my location on the planet had shifted, and my home seemed to be drifting somewhere between where I'd been and where I would be for these next many months.

The nagging ache whenever I thought about my San Francisco life continued. No regular, routine interactions with close friends and nothing resembling a romantic interest gave a curious emptiness to my days. *How long has it been since I was without a man in my life?* I wondered. Since college there had always been someone. Bill, for all those years. And in San Francisco, I knew exactly who I was: a young professional woman with friends, admirers, an active social life, an interesting job, a family who loved me. Here, there were none of those anchors to my identity, no reference point for my existence. That past was far away, on the other side of the world, and I was starting a life that I knew nothing about.

Homesickness wasn't the only thing that troubled me. As the next two weeks went by, my sense of the contradictions of my situation in Kathmandu grew. I passed through the neighborhoods as an outsider, entirely isolated from the life I was seeing. I could see, smell, and hear another world out there. I rode through streets teeming with dogs, kids, goats, rickshaws, women in saris, cows, holy men, and taxis. I could even buy items at the little shops, have tea in the teahouses, and visit the temples, but I had no experience of the people's lives. My own took place in two little cocoons: a lovely gated home that housed others like me and a classroom with guides who were themselves set apart by class and caste.

As the days went by, I lamented that I was just a tourist in this exotic place, with nothing to offer but my gawking eyes and hopeful smiles.

Chapter 3
Getting to Gorkha

After three weeks in Kathmandu, I was about to learn what to expect from the next seventeen months.

I woke in what was surely the middle of the night to a buzzing alarm, and quickly switched it off. The Kathmandu house was dead still and dark, with no moonlight and barely any illumination in my room from the street outside. I lay quietly for a moment, envisioning what lay ahead that day—a drive on the Kathmandu–Pokhara highway, a hike through quaint Nepali villages, seeing them for the first time. And then, arriving at my new home at our field base in the district capital, Gorkha Bazaar. Even the name given the main village of the district was intriguing—a bazaar!

I pulled myself out of bed. By 4:00 a.m. I had downed a piece of toast and a cup of tea, stowed the sack lunch the cook had made for me in my daypack, and was waiting by the door with my duffel bag. Peering outside, I saw the bright yellow Foundation car pulling through the gate, opened by a sleepy guard. A Nepali man got out of the car and started up the steps toward me. It was Gopal, one of the staff whom I'd met briefly when I first arrived.

"Good morning, Memsaab," he said with a shy smile. "Everything ready?" Gopal was of average height for a Nepali, shorter than me, with a solid build and a friendly, open face. Though his English was limited, his essential good nature was clear, and I trusted him right away.

"*Tik chha*," I answered, in a bit of Nepali that I was comfortable using. *It's good.* We loaded up my luggage as well as several other bags of supplies that the field team had ordered. Gopal introduced the driver, Sudarshan, sat down beside him, and we set out through the dark and mostly deserted streets. I quickly drifted off to sleep stretched out behind them, with my head propped against my duffel bag in one corner.

Within half an hour I was jolted awake. Ahead, the headlights bounced up and down on massive ruts in the road—was this a highway? We moved slowly over a few more jarring bumps, and the pavement smoothed out again. The guys continued to chat quietly in rapid Nepali, unconcerned. I slipped back into a light sleep, only to be awakened again soon afterwards. This time the problem was a huge washout that required a careful detour along a dirt path that was harrowingly close to a steep drop-off on the right. The sun was beginning to brighten the steep hills around us, and I had a sudden glimpse of the Trisuli River far below. Frighteningly far below.

We spent the next two hours weaving in and out of ruts, potholes, and washouts. As the day brightened further, we passed a series of small, sad-looking villages along the road, ramshackle buildings with rusted metal roofs and huge randomly placed piles of trash. Goats and the occasional cow ambled about, and tired-looking women in faded clothing looked up with inscrutable expressions at the passing cars. *Who are they?* I wondered. *How do they feel about living in this place?* These certainly weren't the quaint Nepali villages of my imagination.

Finally, we stopped at one of the towns. A dilapidated road sign said "Khaireni" in Nepali and English. The car pulled off the road, Sudarshan honked the horn, and I watched curiously as a swarm of men rushed out from a small building and approached our car. They represented a wide range of ages, but otherwise were all of wiry build, wearing faded shorts, short-sleeved shirts, and rubber thong sandals.

Gopal looked back at me and smiled reassuringly. "Porters," he said. He seemed to know one of the men who came up to us. He introduced him to me, "Tek Bahadur. Our porter." We exchanged namastes, and after some discussion Gopal hired three additional porters to carry the program supplies and travel with me for the day.

The highway we'd been on passed along the southern edge of Gorkha District. I knew there were no roads within the district, only trails on which porters carried everything that was brought in from the outside. And that meant absolutely everything that wasn't grown or made locally: appliances, building materials, furniture, food, clothing or fabric to make it, kerosene—everything. Men who made their living as porters would gather every morning at the main bus or truck stops along the highway and hire on to transport goods in their wicker *dokos*, the cone-shaped baskets held in place on their backs with a woven tumpline. For a day's work they would typically get 25 rupees, about $2 in US money, to cart their eighty- to one hundred-pound loads up and down the hills to their destinations. Later I was to query how our half-size vaccine refrigerator made it to the office, and the answer was: "Man Bahadur, our porter, carried it in." *Bahadur* means "brave" in Nepali, and I had to agree it was a fitting description of these men. I was duly impressed with the porters from the beginning, and even more so by the end of that long and arduous day.

After everyone was loaded up, including me with my pitifully small light-green REI daypack, a farewell gift from friends in San Francisco. I said goodbye to Gopal and Sudarshan and set off behind the porters towards a long suspension bridge that hung down over the fast-flowing Trisuli River. We filed across on the wooden slats that made up the base of the bridge. Protected from falling off by closely spaced wires suspended from cables along either side, I knew it was safe, but those thin metal lines looked frighteningly insubstantial. On that first crossing, I flashed on scenes from adventure movies, where the bridge snaps in two and unsuspecting travelers are flung into the river far below. The bridge swayed slightly, some boards feeling more solid than others to my unsteady gait. I was happy to get to the opposite side, on terra firma again.

We approached a small settlement with thatched-roof houses that fit my image of what the villages would look like. A stray goat wandered through the tiny yards around the houses.

Tek glanced back and asked, "*Tik chha,* Memsaab?" *Everything okay?*

I smiled cheerily and replied, "*Tik chha!*" and we proceeded down the trail.

Tek was middle-aged, I thought in his late forties, with features that looked more East Asian than other ethnic groups I'd encountered in Kathmandu. He was small of stature but stronger than his size indicated, with leg muscles showing under his shorts that looked rock-hard. The *doko* on his back was heavy with rice and other supplies for the team, as well as my personal things, yet he bounced lightly along up the trail as if it were a hot-air balloon instead of ballast.

Our starting point was at an altitude of around thirteen hundred feet, as far I could tell from trekking maps. For the first hour or so I was energized, invigorated by the piercing blue skies, the wafting of unfamiliar green scents from the shrubs and trees that lined the trail, the exquisite stillness broken only by the calls of birds and the sound of our footsteps on the rocky path. The trail we followed was relatively flat along a small valley, with the river some distance off on one side and hills on the other. We passed occasional small houses, stone or brick, with thatched roofs and surrounded by low fences of undetermined construction. No inhabitants were visible. Fields of corn and another grain I didn't recognize took up every possible square yard of soil, butting up against the small yards and sometimes the trail edge.

I was curious where the families who lived here might be, and ventured a question to Tek, who was careful to stay near me while the other porters went out of sight ahead.

"*Manche-haru, kahaa chan?*" I asked. *Where are the people?*

Tek seemed eager to explain, beginning with some simple words I understood—they are in the fields, working. Then he began to expand on that answer, and I found myself frowning and shaking my head in confusion, wondering if I'd ever feel comfortable in this new language.

The pleasant walk in the countryside, with its idyllic scenes and the anticipation of seeing my new home at the end, lasted about an hour. Then the trail began to climb steadily, and what followed was an ordeal that I was later to remember primarily for the horror of it. *What was I thinking? Why did I ever imagine I could do this?* At times that despairing thought was twinned with indignation: *And why didn't anyone tell me what this trek would be like?*

The cool breezes when we started had been pleasant, but by mid-morning a wickedly hot sun burned down relentlessly, step after painful step. I was quickly winded, gasping for breath on the now steeply rising slopes. We rested regularly, often at a *chautara,* a locally established rest stop consisting of a stone base built around large shady trees. At first the pauses were welcome, but eventually they simply meant that every minute we rested meant that this ordeal would take even longer. *Gawd, how much longer?* I asked myself over and over.

Tek looked back at me after a particularly difficult stretch and, noting my flushed face and pained expression, said in English, "Memsaab, tea drinking soon."

After a lengthy uphill patch, the porters suddenly pulled up and dropped their loads against a tree. Across the trail I could see a woman in a small hut looking up at us expectantly, squatting in front of some cooking utensils.

We walked over to the hut, and I was ushered onto a straw mat on the floor. I sank onto it with my pack beside me, wondering if I would ever be able to get up again. We had only been walking for three hours, but I felt I couldn't move another step. I looked over at the woman preparing the tea, who seemed too shy to look at any of us. Her dark hair hung loose, and she wore a long floridly patterned skirt with glass bangles on both wrists.

On the back wall of the hut were shelves with simple consumables—matches, cookies, and local tangerines. The stove was made of brick smoothed over with plaster (I later found out that most of the "plaster" I saw was a mix of local clay and cow dung). It was fitted with two large openings, one for a wok and the other for a large teakettle. She passed out ribbed glasses of strong, sweet tea to each of us, as well as small packages of cookies labeled in both Nepali and English: Glucose Biscuits.

Tea breaks, it turned out, were an important trekking amenity, particularly for porters, who were carrying loads over these selfsame trails that were so heavy I could barely lift them. Teahouses, strategically placed along the main trail, provided both a rest and the energy spurt from the tea and sugar.

When we set out again, I felt a slight boost of energy, hoping that the rest of the day wouldn't be so arduous. For the next hour or so we descended from this first (and I hoped last) mountain, and then I had a new challenge: my overtaxed leg muscles threatened to give out going downhill.

The sun was in full force by then, and the endless trail with its ups and downs continued to roll out before us. We passed occasional small huts, water buffaloes, and scrawny-looking cows, some with calves. They all seemed to be wandering loose without fences.

Gradually, I lost all interest in the scenes around me; my attention was focused on the trail, and on thoughts of getting to our destination. Sweat rolled off my forehead and down my back, caking my neck. I sipped water from my canteen and noticed that it was getting low. My heart raced as if I were sprinting, my face beet-red from the exertion. With each downhill slope came the faint hope: Maybe we're getting close. But hour after endless hour, we just kept going. Ahead of me I watched the porters cruise along as if unaffected by the difference between up and down, rough and calloused heels slapping against their thin sandals with each step.

At a rest stop, I finally swallowed my pride, looked at Tek, and asked in what I hoped was a matter-of-fact voice, "*Gorkha—najik chha?*" *Is Gorkha near?*

His response was not reassuring. "*Tik chha, bistaari bistaari jaanuhos.*" *It's fine, just go slowly.*

Fine? I wanted to snap at him that no, I was not fine, but that seemed pointless. I filed along behind the team once again under an ever-hotter sun. I looked at my watch. We had started walking at 7:30 and it was now 2:15. Nearly seven hours, and no end in sight. I vaguely remembered hearing it was an eight-hour trek (*why didn't I pay attention to that little detail?*). Maybe we were getting close.

Suddenly there was a wide river directly in front of us that appeared fast-flowing but shallow. The path veered off to the left along the river, but Tek indicated that we would cross the river instead. The porters removed their flip-flops at the water's edge, so I slipped off my tennis shoes and socks and thrust them into my pack.

Tek motioned for me to take his hand. It was solid, reassuring, and we cautiously edged out onto the smooth rocks of the river bottom. The water was cold and the current strong, so I was happy to have a steady hand as we worked our way across. The river, as it turned out, was considered safe to cross before the rainy season began while the water level was low, only coming up to my knees. Within a few months it would be a treacherously high torrent, so the only option for crossing it would be a bridge upriver that required a detour of over an hour. Porters were known to have been swept downstream when they inaccurately estimated the depth and current, too anxious to save that one hour.

We all crossed without incident. At the other side I let my feet dry for a moment in the sun, then slipped my shoes and socks back on. A deep breath! Surely, we were almost there at that point. I looked at Tek and he gave a faint smile, looked ahead towards where the trail wound away from the river, and then raised his eyes and pointed with his chin to an imaginary point far, far above us.

"Gorkha," he said. "*Pahile, ukaalo.*" First, we go up.

And for the next three hours, we indeed went steadily up. This was the notorious Cheppetar Hill. By then my water bottle was empty, and I'd been told that the local water was likely too contaminated to risk drinking. Every muscle in my body told me: *You cannot do this any longer!* I began to feel lightheaded, slightly nauseated, and walked more and more slowly, stopping sometimes every five minutes to rest at the large boulders that lined the trail. Tek stayed within sight and repeated the "slowly, slowly" mantra when I stopped for too long a stretch. The porters again quickly outpaced me, all but Tek moving ahead and out of sight.

It was impossible to tell what lay more than a hundred feet ahead on the rocky trail, as it twisted and turned up and over each rise. Over and over my heart skipped a beat as we approached what seemed to be a peak, a destination, then sank again as I realized yet another ascent lay ahead.

Gorkha sits at around four thousand feet above sea level. My best guess, looking at topological maps, was that the hill I had just trudged up involved a gain in elevation of about two thousand feet from the bottom to the top. That would be considered reasonable for seasoned hikers, not out of the ordinary, though a slope of that height would be called a mountain in the US. In Nepal, flanked by the massive Himalaya reaching five times that height, they were just the "foothills." And for me, at the end of an exhausting day, with no previous conditioning save jogging in Golden Gate Park (no hills there), it was torture, plain and simple.

Eventually, of course, we arrived. A few houses came into view, the path leveled out, and more houses lined the trail, some on the upper side of the slope we were traversing, some on the downhill side. Finally, a two-story concrete house with a stone wall enclosing the yard came into view. Flowers peeked over the rocky edge and a small yellow sign identifying the Foundation hung on the porch. Tek grinned at me and pointed with his chin at the house—a gesture that I realized was preferred here over pointing at anything with a finger.

"Office," he said. I looked at my watch. It was 5:30, ten hours since leaving Khaireni.

We went through the gate, and a smiling woman in a blue sari and bright-blue apron met us at the main door. "Namaste, Memsaab!" she chirped. "*Kasto chha? Taakyo?*" *How are you? Tired?*

I tried to smile in response, nodding in assent. Yes, tired would be the word. Tek and the other porters were already on their way out through the gate, after dropping off my duffel bag and the supplies. I turned to thank them as they filed out of the yard. "*Bholi betolaau,* Memsaab," I heard from Tek as he closed the gate. Only later did I realize that he'd said, "See you tomorrow."

Collapsing onto a wooden chair on the open porch, I could see the housekeeper—unnamed at that point—setting out food on a small table in a dark central room inside. I sat in blissful peace, looking out at a spectacular view: a deep terraced valley sprinkled with clusters of trees and thatched-roof houses. In the distance were high foothills, and far off and down to the right a winding river. Nothing marred the pristine beauty of the scene—no electricity or telephone lines, no roads, no industrial structures. I could have been looking at a stylized painting of some idyllic world.

The housekeeper brought me a tall plastic glass of water from a large ceramic filter that sat on a side table and indicated that my dinner was ready. At first reluctant to move, the inviting smell of curried chicken soon had me moving towards the table. Suddenly hungry, I realized that I was already starting to feel human again. I hadn't even looked at the sack lunch I had carried all day.

As soon as I'd finished eating, the woman returned. Embarrassed that she was still just an anonymous "housekeeper" to me, I asked her name.

"Gannu, Memsaab," she replied. She then ushered me up a wooden stairway to the second floor and my small corner room. It had windows on two sides, the floor consisting of packed earth over a rough wood base. The single bed was incredibly inviting. She pointed out the window to an outhouse in the yard, with a comment I didn't understand, and I nodded. *Yes, I'd better do that,* I thought, *and then get to bed.*

As Gannu left the room, she said brightly in clearly enunciated Nepali, "Tomorrow you go at 8:00 a.m. to Phugel."

I was aghast. NO! I absolutely had to have a few days' rest, to settle into my room and look around this little bazaar town that was to be my home.

"*Bholi?*" I asked plaintively. *Tomorrow?*

"Tomorrow. Corinne Memsaab says you go," she answered decisively. Corinne was the project leader, the other American nurse I was joining in the field. Obviously this was an expectation around which I had no choice.

Gannu left for the night, and I sank back onto the bed, disconsolate, sensing that this life was defeating me before it had even truly begun.

Looking back on that first day, and in fact those first few months in Gorkha, I'm astounded at my thinking that I could "trek in Nepal" with no preparation or conditioning, and that I would embark on a life-altering undertaking in such blissful ignorance of what it would involve. But maybe it was for the best. If I'd known what I'd go through that day and for the following weeks, I may not have agreed so eagerly in that San Francisco office.

I decided to take a quick tour around the house before turning in. Retrieving a flashlight from my duffel bag (there was clearly no electricity here), I went back down the stairs and nosed around. The floor on the main level was concrete and reasonably clean. There were four rooms around the center hall that seemed to be mostly for storage. One room held a half-size refrigerator with an array of vaccines and medicines. Nothing looked like a food or a kitchen, though. I poked my head out the back door that opened onto the yard. To my right, on a chair up against the wall, I could make out the small outline of our *chowkidar,* the security guard, snoring softly. To my left was another door.

Ah, the kitchen? I went in cautiously and shone my flashlight around the relatively small space. A faint odor of decaying food accosted me. The shadowy room had a dirt floor, one small high window, a gas burner sitting on a concrete bench, a few shelves that were mostly empty, and a large concrete utility-style sink that, at least in the gloom of the flashlight, looked coated with mold. A slimy-looking sponge sat along the edge of the sink, along with various filthy rags and a cake of much-used soap.

My horror at the thought of ever cooking food there, or even consuming food that had been prepared in that room, was exceeded only by my exhaustion. I left the room in disgust, found my way to the outhouse, and then stumbled back to my bedroom, grateful for the oblivion of quickly arriving sleep.

Chapter 4

The Feast

I scanned the trees on the rise above me to see if the trail showed any sign of leveling off. *Please, lord, let it be soon.* My Catholic upbringing showed up at the strangest times. But no, the only thing in sight was more of the steep rocky trail. The glare of the sun was mercifully filtered by the occasional trees we passed under. But the heat of the afternoon, combined with my own internal combustion, made every passing hour more miserable. Yet again.

"*Kati bakichha?*" I asked Tek, who was accompanying me again. *How much longer?* I could hear the whine in my voice. The day, seven hours' worth at this point, had been an endless blur of climbing, climbing, climbing up the rocky trails, then a few minutes of going level or downhill where I could catch my breath. Then more climbing. Even shaded by my big black trekking umbrella, my face was deeply flushed from the exertion and heat, and sweat poured down my neck and back. Every time I extended my leg to take another step, I wondered how I could possibly keep staggering on for another hour, another minute.

"*Aipugyo*, Memsaab," Tek replied, in a kindly effort to comfort me—*We're arriving*, meaning at the camp where my health team was based for the night. But I recognized that false assurance from the final hours of yesterday's trek. I nodded my head the Nepali ear-to-shoulder way and steeled myself to continue.

Eventually the path leveled off, with signs of a settlement ahead. Suddenly I was a bit less exhausted, with a faint edge of curiosity about what I would find. We were at the top of a sloping ridge, with hills dropping off gently on both sides. Ahead, small fields enclosed by overgrown stone fences bordered the trail, and beyond it lay the hamlet of Phugel, consisting of a few stone-walled, thatched-roof buildings. Walking paths spidered out in different directions from the village, leading to more houses. I was suddenly in a charming fairy-tale scene, a picture from some book of my childhood.

Behind one of the buildings sat a small bright-blue tent and near it a larger dull-green one. A small goat was grazing nearby, and chickens scurried about as we approached. I could see local men milling about, but no sign of Corinne.

A small group of children gathered around as we drew nearer the buildings, peering at me as if to discern what manner of being I might be. They were school-aged kids, both girls and boys, several of whom carried a younger child on their hip. A few shouted "Hallo!" but most were silent, smiling shyly and watching my every move.

I smiled back weakly, wondering how I must look to them—a tall, pale-skinned, light brown–haired woman, wearing a below-the-knee denim skirt, a T-shirt, and tennis shoes. Very different from the small dark-skinned mothers I could see lingering near their doorways, who all wore the same full-length skirt held in place with a bulky sash tied many times around the waist.

"Corinne?" I asked Tek. Just a word, an inquisitive look, was safer than venturing into a full sentence in my as-yet limited Nepali.

After conferring with one of the men, Tek returned with a few simple Nepali words. "Corinne working, coming later." He used that louder than normal voice, the one that we all use for people with language issues, assuming that shouting will be more effective than speaking at a normal level. *After three weeks in full-time language training, I should be better than this*, I thought.

I looked around at the buildings and realized that I had no idea what to do next. My Nepali was not yet fluent enough to allow me to sit and chat with anyone, even about simple things like the weather or their health or their children. Besides, I wanted nothing more than to retreat from this world, rest my rubbery legs, and go away from the relentless onslaught of strangeness that so exhausted me.

I glanced around nervously, looking for a place of respite. Ah, that would be a tent. I looked at them with longing and glanced over at Tek. He seemed to hear my unasked question, indicating that yes, the larger green one was for Corinne and me, and I should go and rest: *arum garnuos*. One important phrase I could remember. He handed me my belongings from the *doko* with a little nod.

I felt an almost ecstatic surge of relief and marched toward the tent. Chickens scattered away from my path. The little goat, tethered to a stake nearby, ignored me. After giving him a little scratch between his horns, I pulled off my dusty tennis shoes, unzipped the opening, and slipped inside. Spreading out my sleeping bag, I arranged my little bag of camping essentials at my head: a few clothes, flashlight, journal, cassette recorder, a book.

"Memsaab?" came a soft male voice. I unzipped the flap and a basin of warm water and a cup of sweet, milky tea appeared. Tea? And I could wash? Too good to believe. I pulled the towel and wash-cloth from my pack, quickly scoured off the day's dust and sweat, and gratefully slurped the tea. Collapsing onto my sleeping bag, I drifted into a deep, dreamless nap.

I was jolted awake with a pounding heart by a high-pitched cry, an unrecognizable shriek. Resisting the urge to go out and investigate, I slowly raised myself onto my elbows and considered my little home away from home. The waning daylight gave the inside of the tent a mossy, secluded feel, but sounds from just outside indicated a commotion very nearby. Mostly men's voices, an occasional shout or barked order, with a background of that universal sound of children playing. I could smell wood smoke, but it wasn't the scent of a fire-place or campfire, more like burning herbs. The result was a reminder that I was getting hungry. *Some things never change*, I thought. *Here I am, somewhere I have never been, never even imagined, with fascinating adventures awaiting, and all I want to do is sleep and eat.*

I took a few deep breaths, somewhat reluctantly unzipped the tent flap, and stepped out. I stopped, stunned, momentarily confused. Directly opposite me, hanging by its forelegs from a building rafter, was the freshly skinned, headless carcass of the little goat I'd seen earlier. The glistening pink body looked at first glance like a some-what deformed child hanging there, arms raised up in supplication: "Lift me up!" Here was the obvious source of my wake-up call.

My entire body slumped a couple of inches, innards shifting, lungs collapsing. Once again I was overwhelmed, defeated by this unpre-dictable life I'd chosen so casually. I knew that killing a goat was a relatively rare event in these dirt-poor hills, only done for special occasions like festivals, or for special guests. The special guest would be me. But that suspended creature looked so gross, so pathetic, that my hunger was completely gone. Like most Americans, I had no desire to see the whole carcass of animal meat I consumed. How could I eat this poor thing? And how could I not?

I slunk back into the tent and waited for Corinne's return.

It was nearly dark when I heard the team coming back into camp. From a distance, the sounds were those of friends anywhere chatting, joking together. I stepped back outside into in the pleasantly cool evening air. Scanning the dim light for the sight of an Anglo face, I realized that I was already yearning to engage in the comfort of casual conversation—in English.

A small group approached the tent, with Corinne in the lead. She was a lively woman about my age—early thirties, I thought—short and trim, with long blonde hair and a charming, direct smile. "Mary Anne! So great to see you here. I thought this day would never come!

Just let us get this equipment put away. . . ." Her voice trailed off as she drifted with the group into the nearby building. I could hear her directing the activity, conversing confidently in Nepali.

Then she returned with the same small troop of our Nepali team in tow. They stood politely in a semicircle as she introduced them.

"Mary Anne, these are our vaccinators, who you'll get to know well. This is Sita Devi, here is Kaliwati, and this is Sushila. And this is Bhim Raj, our wonderful cook, Mek Bahadur, one of our porters," followed by a list of names for three other porters that I knew I would forget immediately. I felt awkward, thinking I should say something polite about looking forward to working with them, but I didn't have the energy or courage to try. They all smiled and namaste'd politely. Ah—that, at least, was something I could do in return: the folded hands and bow of the head. It was a lovely, touching gesture of the Nepali culture, and I would soon find my hands automatically rising into that gesture for any greeting.

Little did I know then how important the vaccinator named Sita would be to this new life I was stepping into. Over the next year, she would be an indispensable interpreter of the culture and trusted friend.

"And this is the *pradhan pancha* and his assistant," continued Corinne, indicating two men who had been lingering near the group. "They've been very helpful in getting the women to bring their kids out for our immunizations today." I namaste'd them too, wondering when I'd be able to actually say something without feeling stupid and awkward. I had no idea what a *pradhan pancha* was, but decided not to ask just then.

The rich cooking scents of rice and curry revived my hunger, and very soon we were ushered through the low doors of the nearby building for dinner. It was the village meeting house, with few amenities but large enough to hold our full team of seven or eight men and women, plus selected village leaders. The walls and floor were smoothly mud-packed, a warm rust color in the shadowy lantern light.

"Here you are, Mary Anne—your first Nepali field meal. I hope you like it!" enthused Corinne with a proud smile. She indicated where I was to sit with the team, everyone cross-legged in a circle on straw mats, and handed each of us white enamel plates and soup spoons. Remembering my introduction to the Nepali style of eating without utensils, I felt a little lurch of gratitude for the spoon.

The cook, Bhim Raj, approached with a huge pot of rice from which he doled out servings to each of us. Next he brought pans of watery black lentils, curried meat, and some kind of yellow vegetable. It smelled exotic, inviting, and delicious. Watching Corinne for hints of what to do (and when to do it), I cautiously dipped my large spoon into the rice, topped with the lentils. So good. Then the vegetable, also quite tasty, some kind of curried squash. Then the meat. That shocking sight of the sacrificial goat carcass flashed before me in grisly detail, but I forced myself to contemplate the room, the assembled group, and took a bite.

The rest of the meal was an unforgettably miserable routine of *chew and swallow, chew and swallow—you can do it, just chew and swallow.* The goat meat was tough, like little pieces of leather—but I didn't want to chew it anyway, because some of the pieces included the slimy, fatty skin, a few with bits of hair still attached. I was revolted. At the same time, I knew that this must be a big treat for the team, a feast. I did my best to smile—hoping I looked appreciative. But mostly it was chew and swallow, just do it.

When we had all finished the meal, Corinne turned to me.

"Why don't you get a head start on some sleep now," she said softly. "I've got to do some stuff with the team." Was she remembering her own first days in the field? It was hard to imagine that she ever felt as inept and unprepared as I did.

I nodded, relieved beyond imagining to be able to retreat to that cozy green tent, a little womb of comfort in this strange, stressful world.

I slid into my sleeping bag, but sleep didn't come right away. Instead, my thoughts drifted back to the luxurious dinner party that was my farewell to the life I left behind in San Francisco—the comforting chatter and well-wishes of friends I loved, everyone joining the hostess to chop and stir, resulting in a gourmet American feast. I was there for a moment, sitting at the dinner table, basking in the warm sense of connection and acceptance. Smooth crystal wine glasses shone like soft stars in the candlelight, and a Mahler symphony played faintly in the background. I loved that life—why had I decided to leave it? And then I was a child again, drifting off to sleep on the rose flowered carpeting on the living room floor at our Montana ranch, as the console radio droned a favorite program, and my father snored softly on his brown recliner armchair above me. I was safe, comfortable, loved.

The sudden metallic din of pans clanging startled me awake. I lay there in the dark listening to the sounds of children's shrieks, a distant radio playing some lively but unfamiliar music, and animal sounds—dogs yelping, the low moans of cattle, the chirping of crickets. Over it all was the murmur of voices, soft enough, far off enough that I couldn't detect the words, the language, just the cadence of storytelling, faint explosions of laughter, the occasional shout at a dog or a child. *Imagine, children up playing this late at night,* I thought . . . and fell back asleep.

Chapter 5
Tragedy in Taklung

Someone was speaking to me from just outside the tent. My wake-up call turned out to be Bhim Raj, the friendly cook. When I opened the tent flap, he passed me a chipped white enamel mug of tea and a basin of warm water, accompanied by the flash of a bright, toothy grin. Bhim Raj was tall for a Nepali man, taller than my five feet eight inches, and already I could sense another difference about him. He wasn't timid around foreigners, the way that most of the porters were. He didn't speak much English but communicated with the few simple words he knew. Over time he was to become a trusted pal.

"Memsaab okay?" he asked. I realized with a faint (very faint) stab of guilt that I had probably slept later than I should have. Corinne, my tentmate, had already gotten up and started the day's organizing. My sleep had been that of a newborn, deep, sunk into another world that was so unlike anything I knew that I didn't even remember it as dreaming, more like bizarre psychedelic travel into another universe. It was suddenly comforting to see the mossy green tent around me, a solid world.

"*Tik chha*," I answered. *I'm fine.* I sipped the milky tea, strong and very sweet, then rushed through some basic ablutions, pulled my shoulder-length hair into a ponytail, and dressed in the same wrap-around denim skirt and T-shirt I had worn the day before. *Standards already slipping*, I lamented. I was ready for the first day of work in Nepal.

But this was nothing like other jobs. It was becoming clear that I'd chosen to live with people so unfamiliar to me that I might have dropped in from another planet. Very few of the village people had ever ridden in a motorized vehicle, seen a movie or television. They had very little money, because they lived largely on what they could grow and make themselves. Awareness of the chasm between my life and theirs, a certainty that I could never have any real connections with them, had begun to fill me with a strange anxiety.

I sighed, took two deep breaths, forced a smile, and stepped into the sunny morning.

We were camped near the *panchayat bhawan*, the village meeting house, a small stone building with a rusty corrugated metal roof. Already the sounds and smells of morning filled the clear, chill air: roosters crowing, dogs yapping in their endless small scuffles, multiple birdsongs that I didn't recognize, and children shouting, with the smoke of cooking fires emanating from every home. Far off in the distance to the northwest, the Annapurna range cut jagged holes into a deep blue sky.

"Namaste, Memsaab!" The customary greeting as I emerged from the tent came from staff members milling about the camp. Corinne gave me a cheerful smile, and we joined the rest of the team in the room where we'd been for the previous night's dinner. We sat again on straw mats on the mud-pack floor, and though the day was bright outside, only a few rays of sunlight streamed in through one window and the open door. Breakfast was a mountain of rice, with lentils on the side and a slice of lemon to add some tang. There was a low murmur of conversation among the Nepali staff, little of which I understood. I ate with relish, suddenly hungry.

As soon as we finished eating, Corinne began directing the preparations for the day's work. Breakfast was whisked away, and all the supplies and equipment that would be needed were laid out helter-skelter on the floor. The porters, I discovered, did more than just their main job of carrying loads, in this district that was fully devoid of any wheeled vehicles. They had other responsibilities, including packing up supplies and immunization cards for the day's travel to outlying villages.

I surveyed the vaccinators. Sita was the youngest of the three women. Tall, I guessed in her late twenties, her intense expression often gave the impression she was confused or angry. Sushila—slightly plump, pretty, and smiling—had a small son who stayed at home with other family members when she was working. Kaliwati was the oldest, a young-looking grandmother who seemed to "mother" the staff. Each of them had long black hair smoothed into a tidy knot at the base of their neck and wore a light-blue cotton sari with royal-blue trim as a uniform.

Decisions were made about who would go where, what was missing, who forgot to restock their carry-bag, and where were the thermometers that had to be included in every cooler to make sure the vaccines didn't spoil. I stood amid the commotion, smiling and trying to look engaged, not sure how much I should be involved and quite aware that my help wasn't needed.

Finally, everything seemed ready, and three teams set out for different villages. Today I would go with Sita and a new porter, Tul Bahadur. My team was to cover the site closest to camp; I felt guiltily grateful for that. We would start with a trek out to the "ward" or hamlet we were responsible for. Each ward had officials who would help us find the children to be immunized and keep track of who showed up and who didn't. If they didn't come to us at a designated immunization site, we would track them down in their homes.

The three of us headed down a well-used trail in the bright sunshine, accompanied by the trill of birds, the smell of cooking fires from the houses we passed, and the gaze of curious villagers who

were already out working in the adjoining fields. The day was beginning to warm up already, but because this was only April and we
were at an elevation of nearly four thousand feet, the temperatures
would not be really hot for another month or more. Soon we started
gently downhill, and though every step downhill meant eventually
one going back up, I enjoyed the sense that I was out for a pleasant
stroll. The trail was mostly through a forested area, so we spent much
of the time in the shade. Even more enjoyable was finding that I was
able to carry on a basic conversation in Nepali with Sita.

"Memsaab, *tapaaiko pariwaar ke ke hunchha*?" Sita asked after
a few minutes on the trail. *Who is your family?* I was to learn very
quickly that family relationships are of paramount importance in
Nepal. Nearly every conversation begins with an inquiry as to the
health or well-being of family members.

"*Baau, Aama, char bahini, duita baai,*" I responded. *My parents,
four younger sisters and two brothers.*

"*Srimaan chhaina?*" she asked. *You don't have a husband?* Now we
were getting into risky territory. In this very traditional society, how
would they react to knowing that I was divorced? Did they even have
divorce in this country? Was I about to disgrace myself if I admitted
my status?

"*Chhaina. Tiyo, tara ahile chhaina,*" I responded. *I had one, but I
don't now.* A brief conversation ensued about the marriage. Did he
leave me? No, I left him. Did we have children? No. Did he drink, was
that the problem? Well, part of it. Have other women? Yes, that too.

Weird, I'm telling her everything! I thought. But they seemed
satisfactory answers, expected, not shocking, and the conversation
moved on to other topics. Sita patiently helped me limp through several topics of conversation in Nepali that day, and I soon realized that
she was going to be the best language teacher I could hope for.

Sita was not your ordinary Nepali woman. She was taller than
most, sturdily built but with the grace that most Nepali women

seemed to have, probably from managing their long skirts, no matter what the activity. Corinne had told me that Sita had been offered an arranged marriage by her parents at an early age, as nearly all young Nepali girls were, and she simply refused. She wanted something besides childbearing and drudgery, the life she saw for most women. Her father, traditional Nepali though he was, somehow recognized that their daughter was not going to yield to the rarely questioned social norm of marriage and procreation. That choice meant Sita had to find a paying job, since she would live with her parents and had to contribute to the household finances. A job with the Foundation meant that not only could she bring in stable monthly pay, most of which would go to her family, but she would have the unique opportunity of meeting new people, seeing new villages within the district. For an enterprising young Nepali woman, it was ideal.

Sita had not actually passed the tenth grade certification required for the job—although she had been able to convince Corinne that she had—but her intelligence and abilities, as well as her unique contributions to the team, were clear by the time that was discovered. Contrary to my initial impression, Sita was outgoing, friendly to anyone we came across, and always ready to poke fun or make a joke. She became our best vaccinator by far, because she enjoyed being with people and talking to the women. There was a kindness about her interactions with the mothers to which they seemed to recognize and respond. Sita would become my window into the culture and way of life of the village women I was about to encounter.

We arrived at our destination after substantially more than the predicted half hour (I already could see a pattern there), a hamlet consisting only of a few scattered houses on either side of the trail. We set up our equipment under a *chautara*.

Before long, women appeared with one or several small children either on their backs or holding their hands. One by one they presented their bright yellow immunization card, on which Tul recorded the day's information indicating that they had received their first injection. Sita intoned a brief, pithy health education message to each small group, and we both gave the injections. The women appeared shy at first, or afraid to look at me directly, but they beamed when I smiled at them and their babies. I noticed two women conversing with Sita and then giggling at something she said.

"Sita, what did they ask you?" I queried, wanting to be in on the joke.

"Oh, Memsaab—these rural people! They asked if you were a man or a woman. You don't dress like women do here."

I was shocked—and felt slightly foolish and humiliated, my femininity questioned. I understood how different physically I was to the Nepali village women—light-haired and at least six inches taller than most. This comment made me see how different I must have looked to them in other ways, very unlike what they identified as "woman" every day of their lives. What I hadn't noticed was that my below-the-knee skirt was similar to the garment that many of the older men wore. The Nepali women all wore a full-length cotton skirt, essentially a large overlapping tube, held in place by a thick cummerbund. Their cotton blouses were all the same style too, with mandarin collars and ties that that crossed in front, no doubt to simplify breastfeeding. Many wore elaborate nose rings of tooled gold that hung down over their upper lips. Some had turbans wrapped around their heads.

I eventually realized that for most villagers, Western women had a kind of gender-free status, performing activities that only men typically did, such as traveling unaccompanied or meeting with village elders. *I must look like a gangly freak to them*, I sighed. *Just one more thing to get used to.*

I had noticed that the women wore a very particular kind of tooled gold earrings.

"Sita, where could I buy some of those earrings that these women wear?" I asked.

"You have to have them made, Memsaab," she replied. "There's someone who does it in Khaireni. You can order them next time you go to Kathmandu." Khaireni was the town on the highway where we started the long trek to Gorkha Bazaar. When, several weeks later, I opened a little plastic bag of twenty-three karat gold–tooled earrings and fastened them into my earlobes, I felt a tiny surge of pride and satisfaction. *Like putting on my first bra,* I thought. Becoming a woman, at least here.

But it was not only appearance and gender roles that set us apart; the poverty of the villages was also sadly apparent. Many of the women wore skirts so tattered and faded that I could hardly recognize the color. Some spoke very little, with an air of resignation about whatever was to happen. Skinny yellow dogs wandered about, looking desperate for the smallest morsel of food. In the hot, dusty day, swarms of flies followed me wherever I went, landing on my ankles and on the faces of the children around me. Though they were beautiful, as children are, most wore ragged, dirty clothes and many had unwiped noses. They clung to their mothers quietly, at least until the dreaded needle came their way, when they screamed in panic.

Everything I saw that day was a wonder to me. This was Asia. This was me, living in Asia, starting work in Asia. I would occasionally flash back to movies I had seen about Americans living in foreign places and wonder how I would appear on the big screen. Not exactly glamorous, with my dusty clothing and so many flies buzzing around my legs that I had to continually do a little shuffle to keep them from biting. I tried not to think I looked like the cattle on our family ranch, battling the same swarms of flies in the summer heat.

After a couple of hours, we had vaccinated all the children who showed up, and that easy downhill trek turned into the part I dreaded, going back uphill. But we'd finished early, so the return to camp was more or less leisurely, and we were shaded from the afternoon sun. Still, by the time we approached the camp, I was feeling sweaty, weak-legged, and craving some of that quiet time that I have always seemed to need: space to go inside my head, to let the "me" inside have a rest. Ah, the tent; there it was. Bliss.

Not quite. As we came closer, I saw a small group of men talking excitedly to Bhim Raj as they watched our approach.

"Memsaab, baby sick," he said in English and then launched into some detail in Nepali, explaining that I needed to go to a neighboring house because a small child was ill, and perhaps I could help. Corinne wouldn't be back in camp for another couple of hours, and by then it would be too dark to go. I missed a few finer points of the explanation, but what needed no translation was the anxiety and sense of helplessness of the men, who it seemed were family members of the sick child. One was the child's father, a very thin older-looking man who had heard that there were *bideshis* (foreigners) in the village, and they no doubt were doctors with medicine (the usual assumption). I started to object, worried that I had no clinical training in either pediatrics or tropical diseases, and I didn't yet have the slightest idea of what medicines we had that might be helpful, even if I could figure out a diagnosis.

But it was a short-lived objection. Clearly no one here knew more medicine than I, so there was little reasonable choice but to do what I could. I scrambled through the bag with the medicines we kept in our tent, shoved a few bottles of antibiotics and a stethoscope into my daypack, and set out with Sita and the men to the baby's house.

Of course, it wasn't exactly in the neighborhood. *Sweet Jesus,* I muttered to myself. *Will I ever believe these people's estimates of time and distance?* After nearly an hour of up and down hills on a small trail, passing a few scattered houses, it was obvious when we reached our destination. Several people, men and women, were milling around a small thatched-roof house just off the trail, and as we drew closer I could see a child about two years old lying on a straw mat on the porch.

Sita whispered, "They are of the Kami caste, Memsaab, so they wait for us outside."

Oh. Kamis were one of the untouchable Hindu castes. People of the higher castes would never enter their homes, so the family was taking precautions, making sure that the sick child was outside their "polluted" house in case help arrived in the form of a higher-caste person. The idea of such discrimination revolted me. But for the moment that concern was overshadowed by the task ahead.

I moved up to the porch, and the crowd moved aside. I sat down beside the little boy, who was very pale, eyes rolled back, breathing in rapid, shallow grunts, and obviously unconscious. One thing nurses learn in working with children, more clearly than all the detailed symptoms or procedures or medicines they memorize, is what a sick child looks like. This was a very sick child. I guessed he wouldn't survive even if we had an ambulance waiting to whisk him away to a pediatric emergency room, lights and sirens announcing the importance of his life, his parents' panic, the neighborhood's care and concern.

And alas, there was only me. I picked up his grubby little-boy hands, felt his swollen abdomen, pinched his skin to look for signs of dehydration, and completed a cursory exam. In my halting Nepali, I asked the boy's father about how and when the illness had started and posed the other usual questions—when he was last awake to eat and drink, had they given him any medicines so far. But nothing in what I saw or heard fit with a specific diagnosis—no diarrhea, no cough, no rash, just a fever and eventually, this.

I realized then that in my ten years as a nurse, I had never faced this situation: Someone was dying, I was the only one who could help, and I had nothing to offer. Waves of something like panic rose in my chest. I struggled to maintain a calm demeanor, aware of many eyes on me. Covering the baby's bare body with a wrinkled cloth that was lying beside him, I took a deep breath and said gravely to the father, "Your baby is very sick."

"Will he die?" was his response.

Before I could answer, I heard Sita say softly, "Memsaab, the mother." A group of women had been inside the house, and I looked up as a small woman, in her late thirties I guessed, worked her way towards me. She was weeping, wiping her eyes with her sleeve, with a look of anguish on her face that combined despair and anger—despair because she didn't have to be told that her child was dying, anger because, as it turned out, this was the second child she had lost.

The distraught woman began wailing a litany of what she had suffered, and even as I wasn't sure I understood the details, I was clear on the sense of it. She moaned that she could not go through this again, she just could not. She had seven children still alive, and that was enough. Was there not something she could do to not have any more? *"Pariwar niyojan"* was a national slogan—plan your family. Could I help her do that? If I couldn't save her baby, couldn't I help her with that one thing, so she would not have more children only to see them die?

But family planning was just a slogan in that district then, and I had nothing to offer. I took the mother's hand, struggling in vain to find the words in Nepali for "I am so sorry," hoping that she could see that I understood her pain. My throat was nearly swelling shut in an effort to hold back my own tears. She continued to cry, more softly now, and went to sit by her small son.

The question asked by the boy's father hung in the air, unanswered. I spoke with him again, wanting the family to understand our concern and sympathy, but that we had no magic to keep the child alive. I had a sudden image of the scene around me: the critically ill patient, the anxious family, the caregiver. I was in the role of the caregiver, but this was a patient who wouldn't be saved.

As Sita and I slowly made our way back up the trail to camp, I struggled to understand what sense I could make of this little boy's death, of his mother's anguish. Part of me wanted to shut it out of my mind, but I knew that these moments would be burned into my memory. What could I do with the misery that I'd just witnessed? Would I see this again and again, and finally be unaffected by it? Should I just accept it, or was there another way?

Much about the scene stayed with me for weeks. I knew that the poverty of rural Nepalis was very close to the worst in the world. But there was more. The cause of the mother's pain was not just lacking the means to buy food, clothes, or medicine, as important as they were. It was having no power over what she could and could not do. She was among the most powerless individuals I could imagine: low in status as a Nepali woman, a member of the lowest possible caste, in one of the poorest countries of the world. She had no control over her life, her choice to reproduce, her ability to keep her children well. In contrast, I was there in Nepal purely because I wanted a change, an adventure. I felt my own privilege shining out from me like an unwanted aura, and it shamed me. She was deprivation, pain, and poverty; I was privilege, wealth, excess. What on earth was I doing here, with my Girl Scout desire to "help people"?

The scene also didn't fit a story line I'd heard about the fatalism of simple rural people: Because so many village children die, they "get used to it." Even the second time around, this mother wasn't used to it. Her family and neighbors didn't accept it as inevitable, and I didn't believe that I ever could, either. As much as I thought I knew of the world, I had just come face to face as never before with its essential unfairness. *No mother should have to see her child die,* I thought. Yes, these things happened, but I had never seen a death that was so unnecessary, so devastatingly unjust. The baby's problem may well have been something that a simple antibiotic at an earlier stage would have cured.

The next day at breakfast we were told that the little boy had died during the night. I was never again called to see a child so close to death, and there was usually no one for families to call in those last desperate hours. I knew, however, that many of the sick children I saw would succumb to causes that could have been easily prevented or treated.

Over the following months more questions arose. How could the village people work so hard, and still have so few material goods to show for it? Why did most of the children look giggly and happy, even though illness seemed rampant and toys nonexistent? Families would sometimes give me small gifts and prepare meals for me—what explained their warm generosity despite such shocking poverty? As time passed, my respect and admiration for the village people I met continued to deepen and grow.

Chapter 6

Monsoons and Mysteries

Torrents, buckets, cats and dogs—none of that captured the density or volume of water falling through the air when the heavens opened up at the beginning of the monsoon rains. It was like standing in a tepid shower fully clothed, drenched within seconds. Then, miraculously, in an hour or two or three, the downpour would disappear, the clouds dissipate, and a glorious bright sun would dry my wet clothes in an odd way, shaped to my body.

It was late May, the monsoons were about to assail us in full force, and I would soon complete my first month of field work. I was anxious to get back to our base in Gorkha village before the onslaught arrived. Many rural projects such as ours would cut back during this time, or even cease activities that required travel. But Corinne had decided that approach would put us too far behind on our immunization plans. Instead, she opted for a three-week break, staying out longer on each trek when we resumed. *A break!* I was elated at the thought of three weeks to get to know Gorkha village better. *My home now,* I reminded myself.

But before the break I had another week of the daily field routine. I went with Sita and my half of the team to Bhokteni, and Corinne branched off with the rest to a neighboring *panchayat. Panchayats* were like counties, with populations of not more than ten or twelve thousand residents scattered around the mountainous countryside.

Given my lack of experience and language skills, I was apprehensive about leading a team. As a young graduate nurse at my first position, I had been quickly placed in charge of the evening shift at a large medical and surgical ward at a busy San Francisco hospital. *In charge?* I had suffered through weeks of stress, near panic, and an extremely steep learning curve. But no major disasters occurred, and no one died. It was a low bar, but still something of a comfort to know I could rise to tough challenges.

A pattern to my field days was already clear: morning ablutions in the tent; breakfast with the team; an early morning trek, usually long, sometimes only a half hour or so, to the day's immunization site; a few hours working in the heat and flies; occasional unexpected treats such as yogurt or popped corn brought by village women; returning home exhausted; and after a *dal bhat* dinner, ending the evening in quiet conversation, reading, or journal writing. On alternate days a runner came from the Gorkha office to bring supplies, frozen cold packs for the vaccine cooler, mail, and usually a welcome note from Corinne on the other team. The system was organized tightly enough that I was at first more a follower than a leader.

Sita stayed with me, ever understanding of what I didn't know and filling me in patiently on the usual practices.

"Memsaab, we try to find out which sites are the hardest to reach from camp to be sure that no one has to take the farthest ones every day," she noted to me in a low voice when I was determining assignments for the day.

Each *panchayat* had nine subunits or wards, so three teams—each made up of a vaccinator and a porter/recorder—would ideally complete the area in three days. Though it was unspoken, I had the sense that if I was to be a genuine team member, I would take the harder to reach areas in my turn as well. *Okay, that's only fair*, I thought, stifling a sigh. I dreaded every uphill battle I fought against the trails.

As we finished the first day's work in Bhokteni, Sita, a new porter named Prem, and I were nearly back in camp when a sudden dense shower battered down on us. By the time we reached shelter, we were drenched. Sita and I scrambled into our tent, and Prem dashed into the cook house, a ramshackle building that served as the village meeting house.

Just as suddenly as it had begun, the rain stopped. I changed into dry clothes and stepped out of the tent, then sat down on a low stone fence at the edge of camp to watch the sunset. We overlooked a vast, peaceful valley, washed over with a soft blue haze. Terraced hillsides rose like slightly rounded giant stairs on either side of me. Dark gray clouds lingered over the horizon, and a massive pink-orange glow rose up above them in the western sky.

I sat, mesmerized by the exquisite picture. The warm breeze was gentle, sometimes fragrant. Crickets chattered, and a mourning dove's plaintive call drifted in from somewhere nearby. I closed my eyes, wanting to absorb the moment, to keep it close by to call on when I needed it. I felt a kind of muted nostalgia, although for what exactly, I wasn't sure.

Of course, this reverie couldn't last. I heard new voices behind me and turned to see a sweet-faced older man coming toward me with three young children clustering around him.

"Can you help, Memsaab? He has a sick child," the village man queried, and then stepped away.

The little family before me was barefoot. The man wore the traditional white cotton shirt, covered by a dark vest, over coarse white cloth wrapped into a knee-length skirt. The two older children looked at me with curious but cautious expressions, hovering close to their grandfather. Though they looked like most of the village children, in need of clean clothes and a bath, my own attempts at fighting the dust and dirt of the villages had shown me what an effort even the most basic hygiene required. The old gentleman held a little girl, a year or two old, tightly against him in his arms. She was a sad sight. Her skin was flaky, her hair a mass of tangles, her abdomen distended, and her little legs and arms pencil-thin. She stared quietly ahead, neither looking around nor crying, the picture of desolation.

The old man spoke very softly, his voice edged with desperation. "This child—when her mother died, she just stopped eating. Nothing I can do will get her to eat. Look at her. She's sick, very sick."

I was overcome at the sight of the despair in the child's face. Addressing him with the respectful term for father, I said, "She looks very sad, *Bau*. When did her mother die? How?"

"Four months past. She had a new baby and got very sick a week after he was born. And then this . . ." He arched his neck back and gritted his teeth, showing me, as no words could, the picture of a death from maternal tetanus. The dreaded "lockjaw." Tetanus vaccine, which we offered women of childbearing age, would have countered this ancient scourge of both mothers and newborns, and prevented the little tragedy that stood in front of me.

"That baby died too, and their father is gone. I'm all they have. I do everything I can," he added, looking around at the small brood, "but what can I do for her?"

There was a weight heavier than lead in my chest as I thought about what this desperate man was going through, and how little we had to offer. The baby was malnourished, dehydrated, and probably had intestinal parasites. There were no services for treating under-nourished children in the district, and even if available, this grand-father would have been hard pressed to get to them. But the little girl was also very depressed, and nothing would bring her mother back. I knew how many small children would die after losing a mother— most rural families didn't have the time or wherewithal to meet the challenge of raising a motherless infant.

I set out to do what little I could, starting with standard talking points about feeding a malnourished child using local foods. Then I gave the grandfather packets of worm medicine for all the children, as well as sachets of rehydration salts for the little girl, and explained how to use them.

"You're doing a good job with these children, but it must be very difficult," I sympathized, as I finished my instructions. The grandfather gave me a sad smile, hesitated as if to say more, then just gave a slight bow and headed off down the trail with the children trailing behind him. *Like little ducklings,* I thought, *following all they have for a mother now. And that baby may just die of sadness.*

I had learned early in my career to suppress the "why" question when facing patients with heartbreaking stories such as this one. But once again I was seeing a new element of tragedy, one that had never been discussed in my training. Here was suffering based on profound poverty, not just disease, and a death that was easily preventable. I didn't grasp then the complicated social and political reasons for this poverty, or why tetanus immunization hadn't been available to the baby's mother. But all the sadness in the world seemed to be right there, around me, that day.

It was a rough week in Bhokteni. My team had the steepest trails, and they all led up to tiny settlements that held only a few kids. I was grateful when Sita suggested that I should take the last day to just attend to sick people.

Everywhere we went we were met with the belief that since we were outsiders—with a *bideshi* or foreigner on the team—we were doctors or at least had medicine that would help. The small local health posts that should have been available for common problems were often closed and, even if open, were frequently out of the most basic medicines and supplies. Though there were frustrating limitations to what I could do medically, sometimes a fairly simple remedy was all that was needed, such as recommending hot compresses and providing antibiotics for a wound infection.

That morning I was greeted with thirty or forty people of all ages, arranged in a sort of free-form line, waiting to get help for their health problems. The ailments began to sound familiar. Many had back pain, no doubt from their heavy work in the fields. A small child had a scalp infection. Diarrhea in the children was a common problem. A surprising number of people had *pissab polchha*—burning urination. By now I knew enough to wonder what kind of folk illness that indicated. Many common symptoms were seen as related to karma, family behaviors, diet, or some other force that I could never figure out. A lot of the new information confused me, made me more aware of my limitations in making sense of it all. It was a relief when the end of the day came, after some successes but also many frustrating questions without real answers.

But the local officials appreciated our efforts. For our last night, the headmaster of the Bhokteni school sent a message that he would like to treat us to a celebratory dinner. At the appointed hour, Sita and I struck out for the school's "office," an annex alongside the main school building, where a long wooden table was set.

"Namaste," Govinda, the headmaster, intoned politely. He was of the Brahmin caste, the highest, and, like many Brahmins, he looked more Caucasian than Asian. He was tall, dressed in the western style of more educated Nepalis, and spoke English well. In deference to both Sita and me, we conversed in a combination of both languages.

The evening was pleasant, with the inevitable curried chicken, a form of rice called *chiura* that was dried and beaten flat, and rice pudding for dessert. As well as, of course, a bottle of the local *raksi* or home-brewed liquor, made of millet and tasting to me like sake. The other predictable element was a flowery speech. Govinda spoke about his gratitude to us for coming to Bhokteni and how long he would remember our presence in his village. I responded in kind—and not insincerely. We had achieved an estimated 90 percent coverage with the basic immunizations, which was much better than usual.

Partway through the evening, a familiar-looking man walked

hesitantly into the room and was ushered into a corner to sit on the floor.

"Who is that?" I whispered to Sita, puzzled for a moment. She answered that it was the *kadwal*, the town crier who went to each hamlet to announce in a booming voice that immunizations were beginning. He was in large part responsible for the strong numbers of immunized kids we could claim.

But . . . why was he sitting in the corner? Then I remembered a comment earlier in the day that he was a Damai, another of the lowest castes. As an untouchable, he could not join people of higher caste at a meal, though it was acceptable for him to sit nearby in a corner. He smiled sweetly when served his food and drink, joining into the laughter with the rest. As we left, I dug a chocolate bar out of my backpack and offered it to him, commenting on how much he had helped that day.

So that's what it means to be an untouchable, I thought as we made our way in the dark back to camp. Kind of like a pet. Appreciated, fed, spoken to. But not quite—human? Here was another painful realization to sink my mind into, when I wasn't fighting for my breath on an uphill trail or racking my brains for how to help someone with a difficult medical problem. Where did this caste thing come from? How did anyone justify the idea that because of an ancient tradition, some people were worthy and others totally not? There were, of course, uncomfortable similarities to the long history of many kinds of racism in the US. But for me, the forces that kept the caste system in place here were totally mysterious. And the bigger question: How should I—or could I—respond, as a total outsider to the system?

No answers, just questions. A bar of chocolate was all I could do that day.

After a rainy night, the day dawned with a sunny vengeance, and we started out on the seven-hour slog back to the Gorkha base. The downpour had provided some relief from the heat, but the slippery red mud it created was also a menace. Our Bhokteni camp had been at the high point of the village, so we started out by heading down a steep path to the main trail. We filed along slowly, allowing the porters with their heavy packs to navigate their way safely. But even at that cautious pace, I felt every muscle tense against the risk of slipping on the greasy-feeling surfaces. Several times I heard someone call out the warning: *"Raato maato, chiplo baato."* *Red mud, a slippery trail.* Not just an idle saying, I realized, after several episodes of near-slapstick skidding and sliding on the slick brick-red surface. My big black trekking umbrella was now most helpful as a walking stick, saving me from falling several times.

At one point I approached a particularly steep, sharp downhill turn in the path and realized that an unexpected skid could send me over the edge to a pile of rocks below. I hesitated and looked around anxiously.

"Tik chha, Memsaab," I heard from close behind me. Bhim Raj was standing off to the side, smiling cheerfully, offering his hand to steady my descent down the trail.

"Tik chha," I answered, relieved. I took his hand and picked my way down. I had already begun to think of the porters as my guardian angels, and Bhim Raj was the best.

We charged on for the rest of the day, stopping under various shelters when the rain came, then moving on to dry out. Like me, the whole team seemed to be looking forward to a break from work. Only later did I find out that the porters, the lowest paid of all the staff, were only compensated for days worked, so they were likely not as elated as I was at the prospect of a break.

Going home, I thought, and suddenly the thought of another home gave a wrenching twist to my innards: with Bill in the first years of our marriage, in a cottage on forty acres, a big garden, a pond, a silence that fed my soul. We harvested sweet green apples from the massive spreading tree I could see from the porch. One still, sparkling winter evening the two of us plowed through thigh-deep snow to cut down a Christmas tree from our own acres. The two dogs we loved, and the cat, raised with the dogs, who seemed to think she was one of them.

The exquisite pain of our long, drawn-out ending always lurked in unexpected places, even here at the top of the world. Charismatic, rebellious Bill was my first deep love. When I realized, finally, that I couldn't live with his drugs, his episodic drinking, his infidelities, I wrenched myself away. Even now, nearly three years after our divorce, I was unable to conjure up that time without a tightening in my throat and a deep sigh.

Roused from my painful musings by a sharp bend in the trail, I looked up, and suddenly we were at the Gorkha house. I greeted the gardener standing at the gate with a smile and namaste, climbed the steps, dropped my daypack, and plopped down on the deeply cushioned chair that overlooked the valley to the west. For now, home.

Chapter 7
Gorkha Life

I'd been lounging on the porch for only a short while when an unfamiliar figure came out from the house to join me, a tall woman with short dark hair and a big smile. "Hi, I'm Kate," she said with the brightest, cheeriest voice I'd heard in a while. She was our new volunteer, here for three months to lighten our field responsibilities.

I was excited. Someone new! In a moment I could see that Kate was energetic and excited to be joining us, having taken leave from her usual work as an airline flight attendant. "I'm really happy to be here and ready to do whatever'll help out," she said. "Nobody has told me exactly what that will be, though."

We continued to chat, and after just a few minutes of soaking in her sunny, outgoing manner, I had a quick realization of how Kate could be my lifesaver: entertaining the villagers. By the end of a long workday, all I wanted was peace and quiet, but local people were— understandably—eager for any interaction possible with the foreigners in their midst.

"If you feel like hanging out with the local people when we're in the villages, that would be great," I said, hesitantly, hoping it would be of interest. "And of course, for me just having a familiar face around to talk about what's going on at home, what you're reading, stuff like that will be fabulous."

"Sounds perfect," she said. "I'm trying to learn Nepali and it would be great to have a chance to use it."

I was elated. We talked on through much of the evening, and I found myself hoping that my fantasy of breaks from being "on stage" at the end of the exhausting days might soon become reality. But first, Kate would join Corinne's team to be oriented to the program.

The next afternoon, Kate had gone out, and I was sitting in my bedroom trying to find a better way to organize my gear, when Corinne charged up the stairs and popped into my room, back from her last trek.

She grinned and gave me a big hug. "Hi! Can you believe we get a whole three weeks to hang out here and just enjoy Gorkha?" She was as excited as I was at the thought of time in the office and the village. We spent the rest of the day in animated chatter about my impressions of Kate, what was happening with staff ("Do you think there's a romance going on in the team that we don't know about?"), news in the last mail delivery from Kathmandu, and plans for our work hiatus.

The next morning the three of us sat out on the porch for breakfast. The day was startlingly bright, with not a cloud in the azure sky. "Hey, for this we stopped our field work?" I joked to Corinne as we looked out at the terraced valley below us.

"Don't worry, if it lasts two hours I'll owe you an ice cream soda," she bantered. A regular topic of conversation was food we craved, and ice cream was high on the list. Though ice cream was supposedly off limits, as it was made from dairy animals that were often infected with tuberculosis, I was a bit skeptical about the risk.

A goal for the break was to spend time with Dr. K. C., the Nepali district doctor at Gorkha Hospital. I had met him briefly and hoped he could help me understand a few of the puzzling medical conditions I'd already come across. Working as a nurse practitioner at my San Francisco clinic was definitely useful, but some of the problems

I saw in Gorkha were new to me, and I had no medical books to consult.

Corinne said she had paperwork to do and needed some time with Kate for orientation, so I set off after breakfast for the fifteen-minute walk through the village to the hospital. Closing the gate and stepping out on the trail beside the house, I inhaled the clean, fresh air, cleared by the previous night's rain from any traces of dust or smells of cooking fires. I felt hopeful, energized, more eager to meet the day head-on than I had since arriving in Gorkha. *Maybe I can do this*, I thought. *I just needed a little break.*

The path soon led me past the local *paani-ko-dhaara*, or water source, which was a stone embankment built into a hillside with three pipes streaming cold spring water onto a rocky floor. A few local women were washing dishes, clothes, and themselves, chattering loudly as they worked. As I approached, two of the women looked at me curiously and said something to the others, and the talking stopped.

I smiled at the group, nodded, and shouted out gaily, "Namaste!" The same greeting came back immediately, equally energetic, accompanied by smiles and curious glances. I charged on, aware that I could stop and try to chat, but my mission was to get to the hospital. I passed the local blacksmith shop, where two men huddled under a low roof with a fire feeding a makeshift forge and a range of hammers strewn about. That humble hut was where many of the metal tools used in this area came from—particularly the long curved knife or *khurpi* that was used for everything from cutting vegetables to harvesting grain.

The trail led on past small thatched-roof houses and open fields, eventually opening onto a very old and decrepit-looking town square. Older men lounged here and there on the stoops of various two-story pagoda-style buildings—a temple, a bank, someone's home—all somewhat randomly arranged behind a stone wall along two sides of the square. Ambling throughout was a mix of chickens, kids, and dogs. A couple of goats slept in the sun.

I was surprised at the sight. This was Gorkha, the ancestral home of the Nepali royal family, birthplace of the nation. It was the capital of what was known as the Gorkha Kingdom until the late 1700s. The ancient royal palace was high on a hill behind our house. Not until the 1930s did the country's name become Nepal, and the capital moved to Kathmandu. I felt a pang of disappointment at the lack of any semblance of grandeur in the center of this historic town.

I went on through the square and down a hilly path to the hospital, which was of solidly constructed stone with a well-kept grassy courtyard, a path lined with hedges, and decorative plants. Dr. K. C., a lean man in a white coat, was just inside the first door I came to, and he greeted me with a deep namaste.

"Mary Anne!" he said with a welcoming smile. "I'm so glad you could find time to come and see us. I was just going to start making rounds on a few hospital patients. Do you want to come with me?"

I agreed enthusiastically.

"I start in the men's ward," he said. We walked into a large room, well-lit by ample windows with half a dozen beds, only three of which were occupied. In one lay a young boy who looked about ten years old with stick-thin arms and legs and a thin, pallid face that could have come from a photo of concentration camp victims. The boy looked up as we approached him, saying something I didn't understand in a weak voice to Dr. K. C. I smiled at him, said a polite namaste, and received a weak nod of the head in return. He was so debilitated he appeared barely able to move.

"How are you today, Ram? Let's have a look," Dr. K. C. commented, as he pulled down the sheet to expose the boy's midsection.

"So, this kid says he was okay until last year, but he's been losing weight since then and has some lumps right here," he said in English, putting my hand on the boy's pathetically thin abdomen. He indeed had a series of knob-like protuberances that were easily felt under the skin. They seemed not to be painful, as his expression didn't change at my touch. "What do you think he has?" he asked.

I looked at Dr. K. C. with what was likely a puzzled expression. I had never seen a patient with these symptoms and started going through the list of possible problems.

"Does he have cancer?" I asked, the only likely diagnosis that came to mind.

Dr. K. C. nodded encouragingly. "If he was in America, that would be a good guess," he said. "But these are lymph nodes, and Ram has a bad case of tuberculosis. It's in the nodes here because he drank milk from a TB-affected cow or water buffalo. A huge problem in Nepal. Have you seen kids with really hard lumps along the sides of their neck? Same thing."

I had indeed seen children with just those signs, rocklike lymph nodes on one or both sides of their necks. My skepticism about the danger of Kathmandu's ice cream quickly dissipated. Dr. K. C. gave Ram an encouraging pat on the shoulder, and we went on to discuss the boy's prognosis and the very widespread problem of TB among his patients. He noted quietly that Ram was being treated, but his condition was so far advanced that the prospects for his full recovery were not strong.

We spent the rest of the morning reviewing each of the hospitalized patients, including those in the adjoining women's and children's ward. One was a woman with severe burns on her arm, whom Dr. K. C. was treating with grafts from the skin on her leg. I was astounded to hear that he removed the paper-thin slices of skin for the graft under local anesthetic with a razor blade, not having a dermatome, the surgical instrument designed for that purpose.

"I just wish I had new blades for each of these patients," he commented, with a hint of wistfulness, when I expressed my admiration at his ingenuity in adapting the skin graft procedure. *Omigod, he has to use old blades,* I thought, vowing to bring him new ones from Kathmandu on my next trip there.

With each patient I learned something useful. My admiration grew for this solo practitioner, meant to serve nearly one hundred thousand people in the district as their only functioning government doctor. I spent time over the next two days with him observing, taking notes, and sorting out the kinds of patients that I should treat myself when possible, and those best sent to him for care.

Over the following months, other Nepalis I came across in the villages showed me countless examples of the same resourcefulness I saw in Dr. K. C. *Need a rope? Just a moment, let me twist one up from some dried reeds we have behind the house. Tired of grinding corn or wheat by hand? We've set up a mill powered by this little stream. Store-bought fabric is pretty expensive, so we just spin and weave cloth from our locally grown cotton or wool from various animals.* The creativity of village people was endlessly impressive.

The rest of the "break" turned out to be mostly work during the day, with Corinne and me sorting and organizing equipment, summarizing vaccine coverage figures, and moving the ghastly kitchen into a clean, brightly lit storage room. Although my fantasies about time to read and relax never materialized, we were at least out of the rain during the day and able to sleep in our own comfortable beds at night. Some evenings were filled with social events: Dr. K. C. and his wife came for dinner, we visited with the neighbors, and we paid a call on Sita and her family in their rambling two-story traditional home.

On the last evening before we were scheduled to resume our village treks, Corinne, Kate, and I sat after dinner on the little porch that looked down on the valley and up again onto terraced hills. It was sunset, and as day sank into the horizon, twinkling flashes of light appeared at houses perched on the slopes. Familiar odors of cooking smoke and curry filled the air. As the breezes grew cooler, I began listening intently to the sounds around us—excited children shouting in play and the swelling chorus of cicadas.

This place was starting to feel like . . . normal life.

Chapter 8
The Black Needle

After the break, we began again trudging from village to village. One morning, Sita and I stood with a small crowd of eight or nine women in the shade of a large peepal tree in the center of a small hamlet. Peepal and banyan trees were never cut down by the villagers because of their status as abodes of the gods. Sheltering branches hung over the edges of the stone-walled *chautara*. The day was clear and bright, with an occasional faint breeze rustling the leaves.

Sita gave the usual description to the onlookers of what would happen as I laid out the syringes, needles, alcohol swabs, vaccines, and a small bowl filled with the hard candy that we gave out after each child's ordeal. She explained to the group of skeptical-looking mothers the diseases that would be prevented by the injection given in the front of the leg (diphtheria, whooping cough, and tetanus, or DPT), and the one just under the skin of the arm (BCG for tuberculosis). They were warned that over the next day the child might have pain at the injection site or a fever and were given paracetamol, an anti-fever tablet, to take if that happened.

The women, stone-faced, moved away from us slightly. They were reluctant to have their children vaccinated, and Sita was trying to wheedle them into doing so. Though I couldn't understand every word, the gist was clear.

"We're here to help your children, to keep them healthy. Our injection will keep some bad diseases away from them," she said. "Why would we want to hurt them? I'm from Gorkha, like you."

The women, each with an infant in her arms or a toddler clinging to her skirts, and sometimes both, huddled together more closely. They looked as if they expected us to swoop in and take their children by force. Sita and I loomed over them, both of us taller by a good six inches than any of mothers in the group. After mutterings from some of the women, Sita turned to me and frowned in frustration.

"Memsaab, they are afraid. Their village chief told them they had to come, but they still don't want their children to have the injections." Her brow furrowed, as if she were half annoyed and half curious.

I was annoyed and curious. "*Kina*, Sita?" *Why*? "What are they afraid of?"

Sita explained what she had been hearing, speaking to me slowly in simple Nepali, knowing I relied on her to fill in the gaps in my growing language skills. "They say two things. One is that they don't want their children stuck with a needle when they aren't even sick." I nodded. An injection, any injection, was often considered the ultimate cure for almost any illness in these villages. However, it made sense that they wouldn't understand why their child should have one if they were totally well.

"But the big problem is that they are afraid of the *kaalo sui*, the black needle," she continued. "Other immunization teams have come, and some have used a black needle. They have heard that a black needle means their child will die or, if they don't die, will not be able to have children when they grow up."

Not that one again. Corinne had recounted the black needle rumor, the result of a previous campaign by a Japanese group to vaccinate against tuberculosis. The team had gone to the villages, as we were doing, using tiny needles for the injection that they sterilized between children by passing them through a flame. Sometimes the process left soot on the needle, turning it black. Since white was the color of purity and holiness for Hindus, black probably meant evil, something scary.

Damn! When I first heard about the black needle rumor, it had seemed like something to file in my journal under "interesting local beliefs." But here I was, face to face with it as a real obstacle. And I'd just spent over two hours on a steep trail to get to this place. I was absolutely not returning to camp having to announce defeat: village women 10, our team 0.

"What should we do?" I asked Sita. "Show them our needles, so they can see that none are black—they're all silver?"

"I'll try," she responded. Pulling out the aluminum tray of sterilized needles, she walked closer to the group and gently lifted the edge of the gauze covering them. *"Hernos ta! Mira! Kaalo hoina,"* she said politely with a coaxing tone. *Look, they're not black.* Several of the women moved up curiously, then jumped back at the sight of the needles.

"I don't know," Sita whispered. "Let's see what they decide."

Annoyed as I was, I also felt a surge of sympathy for the women and their fears. Who could blame them? The primary goal of every Nepali couple was to have children—lots of them—so sterility was the worst imaginable fate. Why risk that disaster by letting mysterious strangers stick needles in their precious children? In fact, massive coercive sterilization programs were underway next door in India at that very point in time. Even though there was little or no written communication between these villages and India, word traveled, probably from returning Nepali men who had gone to India for short-term work. As with so many other fears, rumors, and beliefs I encountered in Gorkha, there was often some logic behind them.

Another obstacle: Most of the conditions we were immunizing against were not recognized here as childhood diseases. Some were fairly rare, though when they occurred, could be fatal. Everyone knew *dadura*—measles—as an important child-killer, but the only measles vaccine available at that time needed to be stored in a freezer. Fat chance of that for us! Our kerosene refrigerator had a small freezer compartment, but since everything had to be transported on the back of a porter, vaccinating against measles was clearly impossible for us. Later, a more heat-stable vaccine would be developed that would save the lives of hundreds of thousands of children around the world.

Sita decided to try one last approach. "Listen. Your chief has told you that this is important for your children," she said sternly. "He would not say this if we were going to hurt them, isn't that right?"

Appealing to the authority of the village chief seemed to move the discussion along. One by one, most of the women came forward with their little ones. We moved quickly, in case any changed their minds. Dil Man, our porter for the day, wrote the child's name and age on a yellow immunization card. After a quick alcohol swab, I placed the BCG vaccine to prevent tuberculosis just under the skin of one shoulder, and Sita gave the DPT shot. They barely had a chance to let out a cry when Sita would snatch a hard candy out of a nearby basket and pop it into their hands, with a smiling, "*Meetaai!*" *Candy!* A very rare treat, guaranteed to distract most of them from their fear and whatever pain remained.

I let out a long exhale of relief when the last mother smiled sweetly and accepted an extra candy for a child at home. By that point, the sun had already begun its westward descent toward the terraced foothills. We said our namastes to the women and packed up to leave.

"Sita, we've only found eight children, after all this walking and waiting," I wailed.

"*Ke garne,* Memsaab?" she replied. "What to do?" was the ubiquitous Nepali response to all manner of hardships and frustrations. It was a reminder of how resigned they had become to the limitations they faced, whether due to poverty, caste, rural isolation, or just plain ignorance of the mysterious forces that shaped their daily realities.

We were scheduled to cover a second site that day, because each was so small. Ah, but small didn't mean easy to get to. We could see the little hamlet of houses that was our destination across a deep valley, but unfortunately we weren't flying with the crows that day. The trail took us down a steep chasm, over an icy mountain stream, then sharply up and over two smaller streams.

At each crossing, I pulled off my tennis shoes to wade across. My wet socks smelled like dishrags that had been used too long. Stepping into the delicious chill of the first stream, I nearly swooned from its icy relief. As I made my way carefully across the gravelly streambed, I looked over with envy at Sita and Dil Man, who like the other Nepali staff trekked in flip-flops. They were, probably, the only option that was affordable for many of them, but so sensible too. In fact, it wasn't long before I switched to rubber sandals most days and saved my tennis shoes for particularly long treks.

As we approached the last crossing, I looked up to see a narrow, but very tall, elegant waterfall ribboning down to the stream. It fell down a rock face, stunted green bushes emerging from the steep walls in unlikely places beside it. The sight was stunning, and I stopped to take it in.

"Sita—look! How beautiful," I said. It was a sight I wanted to engrave in my mind, beauty that I longed to sit still for and contemplate, bathe in, dream under. Sita gave a Nepali shoulder-to-shoulder nod and a satisfied smile. Though we were far from Gorkha village where she lived, this, too, was her home. She was pleased at my enjoyment, having heard my moans and complaints about the difficulties of this life. We crossed the stream just below the falls. The water was cold, invigorating, not like the rice paddy runoff we occasionally waded through.

After more climbing on a trail so steep I had to grasp at bushes to keep from slipping back, we arrived at the last hamlet. It was the home of the local *satache*, the ward secretary, who would help us round up the remaining eligible children. At least that was the plan.

He greeted us warmly with a smile and a deep namaste. An older man with thick gray hair, he wore traditional men's clothing: a short wrapped skirt, a dark vest, and a *topi,* the Nepali cloth hat. Though he had sent out word that we were coming, his efforts were less effective than Sita's had been. A few villagers gathered around to see these visiting strangers, but the few children in sight were sick, mostly with bad coughs. We didn't vaccinate obviously sick kids because of the danger that the cough might get worse and then be thought a result of the immunization, whether true or not.

The three of us sat down on the porch of the house, waiting for more children to arrive. I looked around at the mostly older women milling nearby. Almost all wore the traditional dress of the Gurungs, maroon blouses with crossover fronts and long skirts with heavy cummerbunds. All had heavy gold-tooled earrings and ornate gold nose rings hanging down over their upper lips.

"Namaste, Didi," I began, addressing the woman nearest me, using the respectful term for an older sister. *"Kasto chha?" How are you?*

She giggled nervously. *Did I say something funny? Look funny?* I wondered. Several of the women murmured to each other and Sita, hearing them, whispered in my ear.

"Memsaab, she said she had never seen someone like you before, with such white skin and blue eyes."

But the ice was broken, and gradually pleasant conversations followed. When I puzzled over a word or phrase (or sometimes a whole unintelligible paragraph), Sita would whisper her translation to me in simpler or more commonly used terms. I learned that the women lived nearby and came because they had heard that a foreigner, a *bideshi,* was coming. Knowing I had traveled a long distance to help them, they were sorry more women weren't bringing their children. They asked about how long I had been in Gorkha, how long I would stay, and how I liked it here. We conversed for some time about everyday topics: their children's school, what was happening on their farms, the weather.

As we continued to wait for at least a few children to arrive for immunizations, two preteen boys who had been lingering near the house saw my camera and came forward bravely to be photographed. One held something small in his hands and, when he raised it to his mouth, I realized he was smoking a homemade cigarette. *He's just a kid!* I thought. The sharp, pungent smell of the smoke wafted toward me. But this was certainly a photo-op, so I obligingly clicked the shutter a few times. The boys smiled proudly, passing the cigarette back and forth.

We waited.

Finally, it became clear that no other children were coming, so we packed up our supplies and set off to return to camp by a route that would pass by the house of the *satache*'s grandchildren. That stop was marginally successful, with three more children vaccinated.

Setting off once again for the return leg of the day's journey, we stopped occasionally to enjoy a view of the far-off mountains, sharp and bright against the late afternoon sky—unexpected during the monsoon season. The air was cooler, a welcome change from the morning heat, but the trail was as much a challenge as ever.

As I plodded up the trail back to camp, I fumed thinking about the roving TB team that had brought on the *kaalo sui* debacle. Of course they thought they were bringing progress and health care to this remote area, feeling good about their efforts. But the *kaalo sui* story showed me so clearly how much community perceptions and perspectives of what outsiders do really, really matter. They matter in spite of the very best intentions and talent and skills, or the sophistication of whoever is trying to help. Over time I would see countless examples of well-meaning efforts that weren't helpful in the long run because they didn't reflect a clear understanding of local realities. Yes, a few cases of tuberculosis were prevented by that earlier effort.

But because of an entrenched fear of that black needle, other children would die from serious illnesses.

When I finally could see the tents rising up on the horizon as we approached camp, I looked at my watch. My little team had spent five hours just walking that day, to and from, up and down, with a measly number of vaccinations completed.

Bone-tired, I yearned for a quiet, restful evening. But before I had the chance to retreat to my tent, I was approached by our new "advance man," Krishna, sporting a cheerful smile.

Krishna's job was to travel ahead of the team to each *panchayat,* where he would meet with the local leaders, delivering formal letters of collaboration from the head of the district authorizing our work. Though he usually didn't travel with the main team, when that work was finished he would join us.

Krishna was in his early twenties with excellent English, a charming manner, and flashy good looks. About my height, he was of a wiry build and consistently wore impeccably clean black trousers and a sparkling white dress shirt. When he coincided with the team in the field, as had happened today, I had the welcome opportunity to carry on an English conversation. Having the advance man in camp also was a lifesaver when I had communication challenges, which happened far too often.

"Mary Anne Didi, how was your day?" he asked.

Yes! He called me Didi! I was overjoyed that Krishna was following through with a recent request I'd made about how I was to be addressed. "Memsaab" was the customary way to address high-status women, either foreign or Nepali. It was a term of respect, but more than anything it signified subservience, harking back to the days of the British Raj, designating those who were of an inestimably higher rank than that of local folk. Sahib or Sa'ab was the high status boss, often white, and his wife the madam or Memsaab.

Nepalis, when speaking within family groups, are addressed by a term indicating their position in the family. The family relationships were complicated—for example, "Rajah Mama" would be a maternal uncle named Rajah, while "Rajah Kaka" would be that uncle on the father's side. I hated being called Memsaab, and when I asked for suggestions, the team all said that Didi, meaning older sister, would be a good alternative. Krishna was the first, but soon most of the staff joined in. Mary Anne Didi I became.

Without waiting for a reply, Krishna announced, "Tonight we should show the cinema. I think the best one is how to care for sick children. We've seen a lot of coughing kids today."

So much for the quiet evening. In addition to immunizations, part of our job was "health education," telling or showing families how to improve the health of their children. For props, we had flip charts on child feeding and a puppet show about preventing intestinal worms. But most popular was "the cinema," a filmstrip of slides shown on a battery-powered projector. The images depicted various health tips for mothers, such as child feeding practices, what to do for a child with fever, and how to prevent dehydration from diarrhea. This would be my first experience with our cinema, and I decided it was worth losing my hard-earned rest for one evening.

As the sun was nearing the horizon and we'd finished the evening *dal bhat*, I began to see whole families drifting in from the surrounding area, milling around a clearing near our camp. They arranged themselves on the ground, some on mats brought from home. Mothers, fathers, adolescents, kids, and even a few elderly—clearly this was an important community event. I guessed that few in the village had ever seen a movie or anything similar. But they had heard about "the cinema" and were filled with anticipation that it had come to their village. There was a sense of excitement even among our staff; we were the all-important outsiders who were bringing this modern wonder directly to these rural people.

A porter hung a white sheet against an outside wall, and I noted a hush as the observers tried to decipher what was happening. Krishna brought out a battery-powered megaphone, conducting the official "testing: one, two" ritual. A few women looked startled at the unexpectedly loud sound. A baby started crying. Anticipation mounted. As the sun dropped behind the mountains, I settled near the projector where I could see both shows—the one on the screen and, more interesting to me, the crowd watching.

Finally, Krishna decided it was dark enough for the program to start. The opening slide showed a healthy-looking mother and a fat, smiling infant. I could hear the crowd letting out small "Ahs," along with, "Look, what a beautiful baby!"

Krishna began shouting out a message with each slide, asking rhetorical questions of the crowd. "So we all want our children to be healthy, don't we? Do we all know how to do that? Are your children always healthy?" I noticed a few women quietly frowning in response: *of course not.*

Each new picture brought new comments from the crowd. Look! Huge people filling an entire wall! They gazed in fascination at pictures of a mother giving her baby a bath in a white enamel dishpan, measuring out salt and sugar into a cup of water as treatment for diarrhea, and breastfeeding a chubby, healthy infant. Though it was getting too dark to see them clearly, the expressions of astonishment on the faces of the women and glee on the part of the children watching were hard to miss. Men and adolescent boys appeared less impressed, but still scrutinized the screen closely.

The crowd watched without a moment of inattention until the final slide, and the projector was turned off. In response to a few cries of "do it again!" Krishna assured the crowd we would be back for another round of immunizations, when we would show it once more. Without anything more to see, the crowd began to disperse.

In fact, only mothers and children were going home, while some of the men and most of the younger people were gathering outside the village hall for a traditional *naach* (dance). A locally-made drum was all that was needed to draw the remaining crowd.

By the time the porters had taken down the screen and stowed the equipment, I could hear the rhythmic beat and singsong melodies of the music of the area. A decision: Should I join the group or succumb to my now even stronger need to retreat to my tent? Aching back, hips, feet. *But isn't this why I'm here?* I thought. *To experience just a corner of their lives, if only for a few moments at a time.*

As I approached the assembly, a small fire at the edge of the group illuminated three young women of Gurung ethnicity who stood up to dance. They began moving in unison, swaying gracefully with intricate hand and finger movements. Even dressed modestly as they were, with the same maroon velvet long-sleeved blouses and full-length skirts as the older women, their movements were playfully sensuous. The drum pulsed on, in a rhythm that was to become familiar: DUM dum-dum-dum-dum; pause; DUM dum-dum-dum-dum. The crowd laughed and chatted quietly, occasionally shouting approval at the dancers.

After twenty minutes of enjoying this second show (was our cinema just the warm-up act?), I finally pleaded fatigue and retreated to the tent. Sita and Kaliwati, my tentmates this trip, both gave me a nod as I left, and I realized they planned to stay up as long as the music continued. Sita was still a relatively young and single Nepali woman. Was she hoping for a flirtation with one of the local young men? Kaliwati, a mother of several children, always enjoyed chatting with other women her age.

I settled onto my sleeping bag in the shadowy lantern light. I was lulled by the beat of the drums and the faint sound of the singing, even knowing it would go on until late hours of the night and make sleep challenging.

Soon my thoughts wandered back to the women I had encountered that day. The world they lived in was unlike any life I'd ever known. I was a time traveler, opening my eyes and finding myself immersed in feudal village life. The women's everyday experiences, yearnings, and opportunities were eons apart from mine. I couldn't fathom what kept them going day after day, what they wanted to accomplish, what made their lives worth living. The distance between us seemed insurmountable. But for a while today, we were just women, sitting around chatting, and learning a little bit about each other.

That brief encounter raised an onslaught of questions for me. How many other millions upon millions of women were born, married, bore children, and died in just these circumstances, the substance of their lives never even imagined by the rest of the world? Based on a whim—my desire for change—I'd stumbled into encountering these unique people in their amazing environment. I hadn't had the slightest understanding of all the through-the-looking-glass experiences this change would provide. Yet already, I could glimpse how differently I would see the world I came from after living for a time in this extraordinary setting.

Chapter 9
Bewildered

Our work didn't only involve immunizations. We also collected stool samples for a survey for intestinal parasites that the lab in Gorkha Bazaar would analyze. On our first day in a new *panchayat*, Sita and Ram lined up mothers with their kids at an open area outside the school, and I solicited stool specimens from a random set of community members who had gathered around the immunization site.

My first prospect was an older man wearing the traditional-style long white shirt, with his lower half clothed in a knee-length wraparound skirt.

Me, proffering a cardboard specimen container, in well-practiced Nepali: "Namaste. We want to check your stool to see if there are any parasites in it. Could you put some in here for the test?"

Man: "My stool . . . ?"

Me: "Yes, your stool." I used the only term I knew for it, one of the most common words in the language: *disaa.*

Man: "*Disaa,* in this," referring to the specimen container, with a look of perplexity mixed with astonishment combined with a slight hint of amusement.

Me, patiently, trying not to sound annoyed: "Yes. Can you do that please? We will take it back to the hospital in Gorkha for the test."

My prospective donor looked at others gathered around for help, muttering something to a younger man that I didn't hear. The answer seemed to confirm what he had heard from me.

Man: "You want *disaa*, Memsaab. In this. For a test . . ." Then after a moment, bewildered, "Now?"

At that point I decided he planned to contribute to the cause, so after explaining that we would be in the camp for two more days, and any time before we left was fine, I moved on to the next candidate. I guessed it was one of the strangest requests the man had ever had. The survey later found, at a final tally, that around 80 percent of the people, most without any particular symptoms, had at least one intestinal parasite, and many of those had two or more different kinds.

The days were beginning to pass faster than I expected. Each week was set apart from the last one primarily by where we were based, and I thought this little village would be a winner. The joys of camping inside a school building, for a start. Sita and I were elated to see it had an intact roof, so the driving rains would not, we hoped, leave us scrambling to cover everything up to keep it dry.

The school was in a lovely site, on a rise overlooking deep valleys on three sides. Outside the schoolroom window to the west was a charming view of a few small thatched-roof houses and a big banana palm, dropping into a deep valley behind the houses. Across the vacant schoolyard in the other direction was an array of flashy orchid-like flowers, bright orange and yellow, nestled into the side of an outbuilding. Behind that, several hundred feet down, rushed a small but turbulent river, after which the mountainside rose immediately back up to acres and acres of steeply terraced fields. At the top of that giant set of stairs was a small village, which would be our next campsite.

The monsoon was in full force now. At the end of the first day as we were finishing our evening meal, a ferocious thunderstorm burst out of the darkening skies. Sita and I said our good nights and retreated quickly to the school, where we cowered in our sleeping bags, hoping the roof would continue to hold back the torrents. Lightning flashed nonstop, followed by overpoweringly loud, penetrating rolls of thunder. I had never been frightened by storms, but this one felt as if I were inside a cannon, volley after volley. I remembered hearing about the high numbers of deaths in India and some parts of Africa from lightning strikes, and the metal roof of the school didn't do anything to comfort me. Eventually the storm moved off into the distance and I began to relax.

Miraculously, the next morning the rain had stopped, but there the miracle ended. The rest of our time there was a tangle of challenges and confusion.

"Mary Anne Didi, we are running out of vaccine. Can you send for more DPT?" This was from Sita, the de facto manager of the vaccinators' supplies. "And we need more cotton balls and paracetamol."

"Prem should bring more tomorrow afternoon. Do we have enough until then?" was my query. If not, I'd have to send one of the porters who should be helping with the vaccinations.

"Maybe just enough for two days, since we aren't having much luck here so far," she replied. I nodded an okay.

As we were about to head out for the day's work, Bhim Raj followed me a few feet down the trail with a question: "Mary Anne Didi, the village chief can't be here on our last day for the dinner. We could invite him for tomorrow night, but the schoolmaster can't come then." Our tradition was to have a special meal on our last day in an area and include one or two prominent village leaders as thanks for their assistance. The problem was that we hadn't really gotten any help from this chief, and we also wanted to include the schoolmaster, who had helped a lot. Trade-offs, compromises.

"What do you think, Bhim Raj?" I asked. He was usually helpful in sorting out local protocol.

"Ah, the chief is the most important man," he replied. "You could have the schoolmaster come to the office sometime when we are back in Gorkha Bazaar, right?" Good strategic planning, I thought. It would be a bigger honor to invite someone to our home/office for a chat.

But at the end of the day, just when I thought things were going smoothly, other problems cropped up. As we were putting away the day's supplies, Kaliwati frowned over the pile of needles we were loading into the pressure cooker to be sterilized and lamented, "Look, these needles are just too old—they aren't sharp any more. I thought we were going to get new ones." Repeated reuse sometimes led to tiny barbs on the end of the needles, and a disturbing scratchy sensation as the needle went in.

"Okay," I sighed. "I'll see if Corinne can get some more from Kathmandu."

Then Mek came in with another concern. "The batteries for the tape player are already dead, so we can't do the worm show here." The "worm show" was a puppet show for children with recorded music about how to avoid getting intestinal worms by washing hands and wearing sandals, very popular with the kids. But most of the size D batteries we needed came from India and were pathetically weak, lasting only a fraction of the time a good battery would. It was painful when they gave out halfway through the show.

"And this kerosene isn't good—the stove won't stay lit," was Bhim Raj's problem. Any kerosene we bought locally was at risk of having been diluted with water or some other substance, so was frustrating to use.

That night, flopping down onto the sleeping bag, my frustration had risen to a near boiling point. I closed my eyes and tried to sort it all out, thinking back to previous jobs I'd held—successfully, I reminded myself. My time as a hospital nurse had been full of moments like these. *Did I let Mrs. B's IV run out? I'm an hour late with giving medicines and this old man is too sick to leave alone.*

Damn, I really have to pee. . . . Some days every minute was a race against time, with the finish line at the end of the day giving little satisfaction as I braced myself for tomorrow's shift.

But here in Nepal I began to realize that despite all the challenges, this team was all I needed to succeed. My best move at first was to ask their advice: *Tapaaiko bichaar ke ho? What do you think?* Sita especially was an amazing colleague, helping me work out reasonable ways to move forward on most problems. I could see that the whole team wanted us to succeed, that my success was theirs too. They were proud of their jobs, this work of bringing health (or the hope of it) to their district.

Eventually, a kind of chaotic order emerged from those first few weeks, and I found I could cope with the routine problems. Little did I realize the greater challenges that lay ahead.

Chapter 10

Never Alone

"Jesus! Sita!" I yelled. "Those kids are following me again. Will you get them out of here?"

I'd begun asking myself daily why I was feeling so low, so irritable, so exhausted. Kate was with my team for a month, a welcome respite from needing to entertain the evening crowds, but even that wasn't making the endless attention, exhaustion, and chaos bearable. The thought of another whole year trekking village to village in this exotic foreign land in a district with no roads and no electricity was starting to sound like torture, not adventure. And I was puzzled at seeing myself change into someone I didn't really know.

That morning before starting the day's work, Kate and I had decided to take a Nepali bath at the local water source, instead of the usual sponge baths in the tent. We rose early, without the usual before-breakfast tea, and found Sita, who joined us. The sun was just clearing the trees, and the birds were singing in full force as we filed along a narrow path out of the camp. After a short distance, we came to a clearing.

Ahead of us, icy spring water poured from an eight-inch square opening in a rocky bank covered with vines and vegetation, protected from view by surrounding bushes. The air was fresh, free of the dusty barnyard smells of the villages. Sunlight sparkled through the trees—enough for warmth, but without the unpleasant feeling that I was in a spotlight. The spot was peaceful, secluded. After the past few weeks of feeling overwhelmed by crowds of people and constant activity, I was elated.

It was the perfect place for Kate and me to practice the public bath ritual, and two local women already at the tap were happy to share their expertise. They demonstrated, we followed. Wrapping a lungi under my arms and around my body, I worked my way out of the clothing underneath it, splashed icy water on my exposed parts, and then washed myself discreetly under the lungi. With every chilling splash on my bare arms, neck, and legs, I could feel the tension lift, my spirits rise. My flip-flops sloshed on the rocky floor, and birdsong filtered down from the trees. Donning clothes again over wet skin under the sarong was a challenge, particularly dealing with zippers. But the joy of feeling cool and clean, at least until the next time I would trudge up and down the trails, was worth it.

We'd nearly finished dressing when I heard childish tittering from the rocks above us. I looked up, startled. Peeking through the bushes was a gaggle of kids ranging from about six to ten years old, delighted with their front-row view of this fascinating curiosity—Kate and me. They shrieked in delight when they noticed I saw them, clearly savoring the excitement. These were the children I'd loved to tease and interact with when I first came to Nepal.

But now, every muscle in my body tensed, and I lost it. I was furious. The momentary sense of peace was gone. *My blood pressure must be sky high*, I thought. *Why in hell can't I get even a minute to myself?* The dull ache at the base of my rib cage was back in a flash. I couldn't believe how angry I was, once again wondering how long I would be able to live like this.

Sita whirled around and gave her best schoolteacher admonitions to the group. "Kids! What are you doing here? You should be home helping your mothers!" They giggled some more, then seeing her serious expression, reluctantly drifted back out of sight.

With a scowl, I threw my washcloth into my bag and stalked back to camp, charging ahead of Kate and Sita. I was too furious to speak, barely able to force down a bit of rice when breakfast was ready.

The teams set out for their immunization sites, with Kate on Sita's team for help with her Nepali skills, and I was left to work in my tent on reports and supply lists in the village building. But I couldn't concentrate on the work and began sobbing to myself quietly in frustration. An ominous black cloak pressed on my whole body, and I didn't know where it came from, how to send it away.

Just then Bhim Raj peeked into the room with a question. He hesitated, then did a double take with a look of concern.

"Mary Anne Didi, what's wrong with your eyes?" he asked. Then, realizing what he was seeing, he gave a quick "Oh," and stepped away, embarrassed.

For the rest of the morning, Bhim Raj was on the alert, running interference with anyone who wanted to talk to me. A stream of people came into camp wanting medicine for a range of ailments, and he was polite but clear: "Come in the afternoon if you need medicine, we will take care of you then. No, you can't see Memsaab now." Everyone seemed to be walking on tiptoes, hoping not to upset me. I was embarrassed at causing a stir, but also grateful for the short stretch of relief from coping with the crowds—and those few minutes to cry alone.

That afternoon was clinic day. Spending the afternoon with sick people was a chance to focus on something new, at least a change from the usual multitasking. I set up a wobbly wooden table and two chairs in a shady spot by the school and asked Ram to have everyone who wanted to be seen form a line. By the time I had gathered up and arranged my record book and bag of medicines, a long queue of men, women, and children of different ages snaked up the main path of the village to my table. Though we were far from the hospital and any well-functioning health facility, it was still shocking to see so many people who had no other options for modern medical care.

The first patient stepped up to my table, an older gentleman wearing the traditional men's clothing and carrying a curved *kurpi*, the ubiquitous multiuse knife, in a sling on his waist.

"Namaste, Bau. *Ke bhayo*?" I asked. *What happened?*

"*Ah, ke bhayo, ke bhayo?*" he said, repeating my question.

I smiled. The perfect answer—I'd asked him what had happened, what was going on, but in this culture he was coming to me to find out what was going on. That was my job, telling him why he was sick. I reminded myself of the importance to Nepalis of understanding the causes of sickness, which was often some kind of external force that disturbed the body's normal balance. The person suffering wants to know where the ailment came from, whether it was eating the wrong food, drinking cold water for a "hot" symptom, or one of many kinds of spiritual or magical causes. Fortunately, they were usually able to accept my prescription for treatment without hearing the answer to that "why am I sick" question, assuming, I imagined, that I knew it and offered an appropriate remedy.

I moved on to asking more about the man's symptoms and why he had come to see me. It turned out that he had been working long days in the field and had a backache. Some aspirin and a little demonstration of good body mechanics was all I could offer. Like work-related problems anywhere, the solution was to change the working conditions, not medicine. Next patient, please.

Kate, who was helping to keep the long line of patients organized, came up to me and whispered that there was a child I should see next, as his father had brought his from a village two full days away. I looked up to see a beautiful little two-year-old (they really were all beautiful, but this one particularly so) dressed in a grubby misbuttoned shirt and nothing else. One forearm was bundled up, elbow to wrist, in well-used rags.

"He was burned, boiling water," the father said, with an anxious glance at his son, who was looking around shyly at the gathered crowds. "Can you help?"

I gave a Nepali nod, told the man what I needed to do, and muttered to Kate, "Ouch. This is going to hurt."

Kate held up one finger in a "wait" gesture and headed for our tent, returning a few minutes later with a satisfied look. She spotted Mek standing nearby. "Mek-ji, want to play?" she asked, and began blowing up a red balloon. When the makeshift ball was ready, they began batting it back and forth.

My little patient was captivated, eyes following the bouncing toy intently, and he barely moved as I gently unwrapped the rags enclosing his arm. I was able to clean up much of the blistered skin, apply a burn cream, and bandage him up without as much as a whimper from the child.

When I was finished, Kate presented the balloon to the little boy. "*Kasto raamro!*" she said to the father. *He's so good!* The man nodded proudly, and after receiving instructions and supplies for the next dressing change, they were on their way home.

Then I was immersed in the sheer effort required to do what I could for all the others waiting: listen patiently to each problem, probe for bits of information, examine where relevant, and decide what if anything could be done—eighty-three times that day. It was a marathon of stomach aches, colds, and backaches as well as a shocking number of really sick people. Two had abscesses, infections with huge painful pouches of pus under the skin, one on a child's scalp and one on a young man's shoulder. Those were the easy problems; I cleaned the skin and with my trusty scalpel lanced the abscesses open. The onlookers gasped at the sight of the pus flowing out freely onto gauze pads. But after instructions to soak the site with a warm wet cloth several times a day, I could send them off with a feeling of having done something useful.

Other problems were not that simple. By the end of the day,

seventeen were sick enough that I advised them to go to Gorkha hospital to see Dr. K. C. They included conditions that I took to be a severe kidney infection, a prolapsed uterus, TB of the spine or Pott's disease, lymphatic TB in the nodes of the neck, severe cataracts, a heart valve abnormality, and several cases of advanced lung disease. Chronic lung disease was a huge problem, since most cooking fires were located inside the main room of the house. With no chimney, the smoke wafted freely about the house until it escaped through the thatched ceiling/roof. As a result, women in particular were constantly exposed to the smoke, which has been estimated as the equivalent of smoking four hundred cigarettes daily.

An older woman was brought on her husband's back, crouched inside a *doko*. After the usual inquiries, I couldn't figure out the cause of her problem, whether it was something serious or just simple constipation. She didn't look really ill, so I sent them home with an edge of guilt that I had so little to offer after all the effort it had taken to carry her to me.

Toward the end of the day, another older woman sat across from me and told me softly that her problem was profuse vaginal discharge and pain. I decided to examine her last, and when the end of the line finally came I beckoned for her to come into the privacy of the schoolhouse for a pelvic exam. She lay back on a bench, smiling weakly, as I gently used my gloved hand to check for anything unusual in her pelvis. What I felt caused me to stifle a gasp. The mass I felt had the consistency of rotten cauliflower, oozing, lumpy, and cancerous. It was accompanied by the pungent, sickening odor of decay.

I withdrew my hand quickly, took in a deep breath and asked her to sit up.

"Aamaa, I think you need to go to the hospital for this problem," I told her. "It won't get better without strong medicine. Can you do that?" I mentioned that the mission hospital on the other side of the

district, which had surgical capacity as well as an adequate supply of
specialty medicines, was the best option.

"Will I get better?" she asked solemnly, as if my words were what
she had expected to hear.

"I don't know," I answered, slowly. "The mission hospital could do
an operation if you need it, and they have medicines too." I held out
a sliver of hope that the problem might have been caused by genital
tuberculosis, not cancer, in which case she could possibly be treated
effectively.

I wrote the names of some locally available painkillers on a slip of
paper that I thought might help control her discomfort. She nodded,
got up from the bench and walked slowly back outside where her
elderly husband was waiting for her.

As I watched the couple walk away, arm in arm, any energy I had
left from the day drained away. I had likely just seen advanced cer-
vical cancer, yet another reproductive health problem that Nepali
women had to endure, with essentially no hope of care. Pap tests for
early identification and treatment of the problem were standard practice in the US and other industrialized countries. Here, it was rarely
identified in time for effective treatment. Certainly not in these rural
areas, where the traditional healer was usually the first care provider
seen, and biomedical treatment would require the totally impossible
trip to Kathmandu.

I've seen a lot of sick people, but it never felt like this, I thought.
Here, I faced not only illness and probable death, but also the links
between life, death, and—once again—the profound injustice of the
conditions of these people's lives.

That night a group of local young people gathered with our porters for an impromptu session of local music and socializing. But I
begged off and retired early, pleading exhaustion from the long day
and intensely grateful that Kate was with me to play the part of the
foreign visitor to the village. It was the perfect opportunity for her

to represent us in a local celebration, which she was delighted to do. Sadly, I knew that her three months with us would be up soon, so having my own goodwill ambassador would be a thing of the past. I retreated to the relative luxury of private "camping" within the four walls of the local school, instead of the steamy confines of a tent, since school was not in session.

For an hour or so I read by the dim lantern light, and then Kate joined me. We settled into our sleeping bags, with the singing and laughter in the background a kind of comforting lullaby. Thoughts of the patients I had seen that day slowly merged into the music, and I knew the blissful, if temporary, amnesia of sleep would soon arrive.

However, a small horde of kids decided that the strangers camped inside the schoolhouse were more interesting than the music, even though there was nothing for them to see through the open, pane-less schoolroom windows. After calling out a few times, they started throwing stones onto the corrugated metal roof, then giggling wildly, hoping for a response.

"Omigod. What do we do about that?" I asked Kate in a whisper.

"You know, let's just ignore them for a while," was Kate's reply in a low voice. "They'll get tired of it pretty soon if we don't give 'em the attention they want."

The noise of each rock was shattering, like an electric shock, but I lay motionless in the dark. I'd always enjoyed the playful spirit of children that seemed to prevail in Nepal, no matter how constrained their circumstances or how few "things" they had. I determined to be tolerant, calm, understanding that they were just having fun. Eventually the noise stopped, and I dropped off into a light slumber.

Suddenly, I was startled awake by a small object landing on my chest with a thump. I shrieked, not sure what was happening in the near-total darkness. Sitting bolt upright, I croaked, "What's happening?"

"Huh?" responded Kate groggily.

Switching on my flashlight, I found the small round rock that had been tossed in by one of the children and had bounced off my chest. Suppressed giggles came from the open windows. Now, I was fully awake and very angry. *I'm going to kill those kids, every single one*, I muttered furiously to myself. With that I bounded out of my sleeping bag and strode to the door, aware that the scrubs I wore for pajamas might look odd but were at least decent.

I threw open the door and could see a small crowd of kids lurking along the windowed side of the building, their grinning little faces full of excitement. Grabbing the first boy I could see by his grubby collar, I charged with him into the middle of the crowd gathered around a fire on the other side of the building. Dozens of eyes turned on me as the music and chattering abruptly stopped, bringing an uneasy silence.

I broke into a frenzied rant in my worse-than-usual Nepali. "These kids are throwing rocks at me! What am I supposed to do? I have to sleep—you need to stop them, right now!" Immediately, everyone was apologizing, scolding the children, and promising me it wouldn't happen again. Dil Man, our youngest porter, emerged from the group.

"Okay, you can go back, we'll make sure they don't bother you anymore," he assured me. But the faintly horrified look on his face told me I had overstepped the bounds of "annoyed" into something most Nepalis were uncomfortable with, particularly from a foreigner—an open display of anger.

I shook my head in disgust, sighed deeply, and returned to the dark schoolroom. Already I could feel my temper slinking off like a chastised puppy, and an oh-no-I-shouldn't-have-done-that feeling rising in my chest.

"Oh geez. It was just those kids, of course," I sighed to Kate. "Damn. I shouldn't have gotten so mad—but sometimes I think I will totally flip out in this place. I don't know how much longer I can take it!"

"Yeah, it can really get to you after a while," Kate murmured sympathetically. But I could tell that she had far more patience for the constant scrutiny than I did.

Knowing that sleep would be slow to return, I sighed and crawled back into my sleeping bag. Losing one's temper is not a good thing in most cultures, but particularly so in this part of South Asia. Maintaining balance, the appearance that all is well within the community, is an important principle of daily interactions.

Five minutes later, the music resumed, but more softly, and the singing continued into the night. I turned, sleepless, from one side to the other, wishing my thin foam pad were a real mattress. I wondered what had happened to the "nice" me, that kind, caring lover of children I'd been when I arrived. Already this life was more frustrating, exhausting, and crazy-making than I could have imagined.

I had never seen that angry, quick-tempered side of myself before. It felt like a mental illness, a total breakdown of the normal person I thought I was, as if some wicked alter ego was taking over. I was at once embarrassed and unable to stop my nasty reactions to regular, daily stresses. When I thought of going on like this for weeks, months into the future, I felt my breathing stop. There was only a dark, heavy space in my chest that wouldn't admit air, wouldn't open to the world.

Being under continuous surveillance was something I hadn't expected, and I'd had no idea how badly I would react. But from the moment we started out on a trek until we got back to our field base, there were always eyes on me. Often it was people telling me their symptoms, asking for help and medicine, waiting for a response. Other times the very novelty of a stranger in the village might warrant a surreptitious trip to our camp in the hope of sighting the foreigner.

Recently I'd started snarling at the first sign of being approached by anyone for health problems unless it was the designated clinic day. The kids had been especially persistent, following me wherever I went and giggling at anything I did or said. As a result, I felt like a hunted animal. Retreating to my tent wasn't an option, as the oppressive heat meant I had to keep the tent flap open. When I did that, a mass of smiling children and curious adults would inevitably gather to stare in at me, muttering to each other at my every move.

Though I was exhausted from hours of trekking every day, it was the lack of privacy that most upset me. Not the heat, the flies, the fleas, the dirt, or eating the same food for every meal. It was that I so rarely had a moment to myself, to retreat from the world, to go into that private place inside me.

I knew about culture shock, but this was a different kind of stress, something more personal. I couldn't even explain it in Nepali since *eklaai*, the Nepali term for "alone," was also the word used for feeling "lonely." Still pondering what my behavior was telling me and what I could do about it, I eventually slipped into a restless sleep.

The next day, I thought guiltily about the previous night, trying again to analyze the sources of my fury. Other Americans doing this work were excited about every aspect of this life, exulting about how amazing it was. Why couldn't I be like them? I wanted to "be here now" too, as the gurus instruct, happily immersed in this fascinating once-in-a-lifetime experience. How could I admit to being such a dull, limited character? It was a guilty secret I could only acknowledge to myself, too ashamed to talk about it or to write about it in my letters home. The feeling that I was failing to fully live this amazing opportunity was a secret burden, and thinking about it made me close my eyes and take a deep breath. I wanted to exhale it out of my life.

Many years later, I heard a lecture describing the introverted personality as someone needing regular time alone, quiet and unstimulated. When introverts don't have that chance to recharge their batteries, they feel anxious and off-balance. And there I was! It had been a perfect setup for making someone like me half crazy: cut off the possibility of alone time; make her the undivided center of attention, surrounded by an unfamiliar culture that values constant social interaction and physically taxing days.

Eventually I learned ways to find the time and space I needed. But years later, on my first visit to a zoo after returning to the States, I found myself looking away uncomfortably from the chattering chimpanzees in the primate cage. *I know how you feel*, I whispered to them as I walked on.

Chapter 11

Festival Time

Though I rarely saw a Western calendar, I could feel the weeks begin to whir by, differentiated only by the names of the villages, the trails, the local officials we met, and our successes (or not) in getting the children vaccinated. We endured the rain, celebrated the moments of sun. Then as late summer approached and the monsoon began to diminish, a mass of festivals began to converge, one after another, every week or two.

One evening at dinner, Krishna reminded the team that the next day was Janai Purnima, the day that high caste Hindu men get their new sacred cords.

"Hooray! Does that mean we get the day off? And what's a sacred cord?" I asked him, smiling expectantly.

"Ah, sorry, but it will only take a little while, first thing in the morning. We'll just start late so Prem and Bharat can have their ceremony with the priest." They were our two high-caste staff members. Krishna explained that the sacred cords are cotton strings that are worn for the whole year under high-caste men's clothing, draped over one shoulder and looped across their chest to the waist. An important symbol, the sacred cord initiates boys into the religion in a lengthy ceremony when they are around six years old.

Prem and Bharat disappeared immediately after breakfast. When they returned soon afterward, Sita, Ram, and I set off for the day's immunization site. We had barely started down the trail when Sita motioned for me to stop. Walking slowly towards us was an older gentleman in voluminous white traditional clothing, carrying a large leaf bowl in one hand and a staff in the other.

"Mary Anne Didi, we can get our sacred cord today too," Sita said to me with a bright smile. "He is a priest."

I gave her a curious look. She explained that middle- and lower-caste Hindus—even non-Hindus—can get a sacred cord, to be worn on the wrist instead of the torso.

I was elated at being able to have a more active part in this fascinating culture, rather than just watch it from the outside. We put down our daypacks and each gave a deep "*Namaskaar*," a more formal and respectful version of namaste, to the priest. I whispered to Sita, "Let me know what I'm supposed to do, okay?"

"You don't really have to do anything," she replied, with one of her quizzical looks which seemed to say: *What would there be to do?*

Sita said a few quick words to the priest, and he put his leaf bowl down onto a nearby rock. Taking one of the cords, he began intoning a repetitive sounding prayer as he wrapped the cord three times around my left wrist and tied it. Next, he plastered a fat lumpy *tika* onto the middle my forehead, a blob of crimson paste mixed with rice grains. I had the vague sense of being at Mass as a child, receiving Holy Communion, and not sure if I was feeling all the reverence I was supposed to.

"His prayers asked that good comes to you, and evil does not," said Sita, as he turned to her and went through the same process. Ram was last, after which the priest picked up his leaf bowl and went on his way down the path.

For the rest of the day and the next, good luck did, in fact, come to me. Everything went incredibly smoothly. I'd had nearly three weeks of sinusitis and a sore throat, which finally cleared up. The work went well too. I felt little of the restlessness and discouragement of the past few weeks and enjoyed a few brilliant days and silver nights. Some evenings when night fell, the Himals would show faintly in the light of the full moon, with fog drifting in and out of the houses and trees along the hills. I did, indeed, feel blessed.

We moved on to the next village, Dhawa, a leisurely six-hour trek away, and Kate left to join Corinne's team. Because the students were on holiday, the local schoolhouse was again available for our campsite. More good luck.

The first morning in Dhawa I woke with a start, squinting at the bright daylight streaming through the schoolroom window. Puzzled, I tried to think why Bhim Raj hadn't greeted me with the usual early morning cup of tea and basin of warm wash water. I couldn't hear any of the expected sounds of the team getting out equipment and vaccines, organizing for the day's work. Then through the unusual quiet, a distant sound of laughter and a squawking horn drifted in with the dust motes, and I remembered: The day was Gai Jatra, the cow festival. The village was celebrating.

Yes! A whole day off! I thought. Days without work when we were in the field were rare, as we had to use every possible opportunity to find kids to vaccinate. But during rice harvest or any really big holiday such as this one, it would be pointless to try to find women home with their small children. I felt a hint of anticipation, a lifting of spirits. To honor the event, I dressed in a new skirt I had bought in Kathmandu, a long wraparound red and gold Indian print, then went out to the breakfast room and found Sita, who had just finished eating.

"Good morning, Sita! You slept well?" I asked, realizing I sounded more cheerful than I had in some time.

"Very well, Mary Anne Didi. You too? You're ready for Gai Jatra?" she inquired.

I knew this was an important holiday. Though I'd already despaired of having any real comprehension of the Hindu religion and customs, I longed to be able to share in the excitement that everyone, old and young, seemed to feel on festival days. *Is it like Thanksgiving, or Christmas without presents?* I wondered. Those days at home were always special, even though I spent very little time recalling their origins.

"Yes, I'm ready! Tell me about it," I replied, as I accepted the plate of rice and dal she politely handed me and sat to begin eating. "What's Gai Jatra about?"

"We're remembering people in our families who died this year," she answered. "You know that cows are gods to us. To make sure the person who died goes on to a better life, we have a procession through the village with our cows."

"Everyone has cows?" I asked.

"Oh, no, they can wear costumes instead. Someone in the family can wear the dress of a cow."

I didn't consider asking why marching through the streets would improve the long-term prospects of their families in the afterlife. Having grown up lighting candles for the repose of the souls of departed Catholics, I understood the yearning to do something to connect with loved ones who were gone, and perhaps even do something to comfort them wherever they were. I wondered if this ritual provided the same sense of sadness and remembering that came with the Memorial Day ritual of placing flowers on the graves of departed family members. Maybe it did.

I ate quickly and we left together down a dusty pathway to the center of the village where the celebration was underway. A mass of villagers milled around, the women wearing their brightest, cleanest outfits: red blouses and cummerbunds over freshly washed, full-length dark skirts. Everything spelled excitement—jostling crowds of people of all ages, shouts of laughter and sounds of animated conversations, among women especially, and meaty, smoky smells from small food concessions.

In the center of an interested circle of onlookers, a group of young men dressed in women's clothing performed a dance mimicking rice planting. They reached down to plant imaginary rice seedlings, then jumped up, then leaned down again in a steady rhythm, accompanied by an impressive band of drums and a horn with the air of a lamenting oboe. In their own worlds of make-believe and fun, kids raced around the edges of the dancing. We walked farther and saw men dancing around in large brightly colored masks, some with horns and evil grins. Were they animals? Devils? The cow costumes were likely among this group, as there were few cattle to be seen.

Raucous laughter erupted from a group watching a character sporting a yellow wig resembling a mop and large floppy boots. He flailed around jerkily, in great contrast to the graceful movements of the other dancers.

"Who is he supposed to be?" I asked Sita. She laughed and looked slightly embarrassed.

"Oh, Mary Anne Didi, he is supposed to be a trekker!" she replied, and gave a guilty-sounding laugh. Trekker, the popular term for tourists sometimes encountered on their trails, had entered the local language. *Oh geez*, I wondered, feeling a flush of embarrassment. I could see that Sita worried that I might be offended. And I was, a little. *Is that how I look to them? So different, so foreign as to be a ridiculous spectacle?*

Another look at the chasm between who I was and who they were, and sadness at that thought. *Will I never be part of this place?* I wondered. My angst-filled adolescence as an outsider, going from a one-room country school to high school in town, haunted me again. No matter who I'd become as an adult, that sense of exclusion, of not belonging, would flash back at the most unexpected times.

I gulped down my pride, smiled bravely at the caricature of the strange-looking, awkward "foreigner," and we moved on down the street.

The crowd surged in one direction or another to see the newest spectacle. I wandered through clumps of people with Sita beside me and thought wistfully that if only I were shorter and darker I could blend in—though I was grateful that, at the moment, other sights seemed more interesting to the villagers than the foreigner in their midst. There was something familiar about the buzz of activity and anticipation that seemed to hang in the air, like a festival anywhere that gives people a chance to stop work and throw off everyday worries. Everyone seemed transported. *This will be fun!* I thought, feeling a twinge of nostalgia for the county fairs of my childhood.

Wanting to capture the spirit of a group of brightly dressed women who were laughing hilariously at the mop-wigged "trekker," I pulled my camera from my daypack. But as soon as I began to set up the picture, one of them noticed what I was doing and shouted at the group. Their laughter stopped as if they had been struck. They turned towards me, standing erect with serious poses, killing the real-life action shots I wanted.

"*Hoina, no*, just keep watching, don't stop," I pleaded.

It was no use. No one in the village owned a camera, and very few even had family pictures. But they knew what I was doing and assumed the only proper pose they knew: solemn, unsmiling. *I can never be an invisible observer*, I thought, sighing, and retired the camera for the day.

Back at our schoolhouse camp that night, we gathered for a special holiday meal that included chicken and extra vegetables. The team joked and laughed more than usual. As soon as the sun set, the heat of the day dissipated and we ambled back to the center of the village to see the *naach*, traditional dancing that was an essential part of any local celebration.

As always, there were impressive village-made drums, some the size of a kettledrum and others smaller. The drumbeat was the same familiar rhythm that I'd heard in other villages. A graceful young woman danced, surrounded by a circle of singers who chanted a repetitive melody. The lyrics included a lot of improvisation, local events woven into song-stories. The dancer bent and swayed to the music, with torso, arms, and wrists flowing in graceful circles as if she were swimming, afloat in a sea of sensuous rhythms. Off to the side, an open fire flickered onto the mud-pack buildings nearby, providing a light show for the crowd of onlookers arranged around the remaining edges of the performers. They crouched on the ground, some on homemade straw mats or low makeshift stools.

I looked up in the faint light to see the teacher from the school where we were camping. He smiled and held out a white enamel cup.

"Would you like some *raksi*, Memsaab?" he asked in his most polite English. I accepted the cup, filled with the local millet-based home brew, nodded my thanks, and he ambled on. The drink had a hint of anise but was otherwise like all the home brew here—clear, watery concoctions, only weakly alcoholic, with a metallic taste that was unfamiliar but not unpleasant.

Just as I began relaxing into the music, explosive shouting came from outside a house nearby the *naach*. The music stopped, and there was more shouting. Bhim Raj rushed up, eyes bright.

"Mary Anne Didi, it's better if you go to bed now," came his surprisingly commanding voice. Bhim Raj was by far the tallest of the porters, and I wondered if he was dispatched to escort me back to the schoolroom for that reason. He was smiling—Bhim Raj smiled readily and often. But there was a kind of controlled urgency in his voice that made me realize something unusual was going on. His tone was one of brotherly concern.

"The men are fighting," whispered Sita, coming up behind me. Alas, it being a festival day, several of the men had indulged in too much *raksi*. A fight had broken out from a long-standing dispute over a local woman, and there were concerns that more violence was possible. *Ah, yes,* I thought, *just like rodeo night at home. Too much beer and celebrating.*

"Mary Anne Didi, I'll sleep with you tonight. You might be afraid to be in there alone," Sita said sweetly, with a look of concern.

I stifled a sigh. Sita's offer was a kind of loving protectiveness, since the worst thing that can happen to a Nepali is to be isolated from others. After a full day of public activities, I was ready to be alone with my lantern and journal for the rest of the night, but we were quickly ushered into my schoolhouse room. The windows were shuttered, the door barred.

"Thank you, Sita," I murmured as we settled into our sleeping bags.

I lay awake for a long time and reminisced about the rural county fair and rodeo of my childhood. Growing up, the fair was second only to Christmas as a time of excited anticipation. My whole family—Mom, Dad, and all six kids—would wander down the main pathway of the fairgrounds together on opening day. We passed through the concrete arch at the entrance and along a row of kiosks featuring custom-monogrammed belts, the best knife sharpener in the country, and cowboy hats guaranteed to last a lifetime. Next came food booths, and then the carnival rides and kiosks. The smorgasbord of familiar and exotic smells, from barbecued meat to cotton candy, combined in a unique aroma that would always "take me to the fair."

Despite the sudden end to the evening's events, I felt comforted, even reassured by the excitement of the villagers, Sita's companionship, and the care I felt from the team when a problem arose. *Maybe I'm getting over my culture shock,* I pondered. *I'm starting to feel at home.* I was making real connections with my Nepali team, and also with this new and exotic place. It was like nowhere I had ever known, but at the same time it was warmly familiar. The initially strange was becoming reassuring, even ordinary. *It's like thinking you're lost,* I thought, *and suddenly realizing that home is right around the corner.*

For perhaps the first time since coming to Gorkha, I had a sense of belonging there, right where I was, doing just what I was doing. *Maybe I'll make it through the year after all,* I mused, as I drifted off.

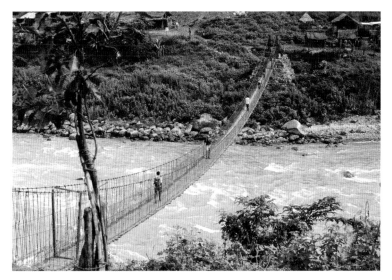

The footbridge at Khaireni, linking Gorkha District to the Kathmandu-Pokhara highway

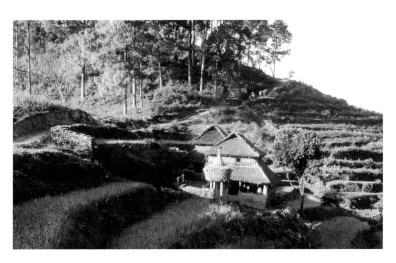

The Gorkha version of a superhighway--the main trail, with porters rounding the hill

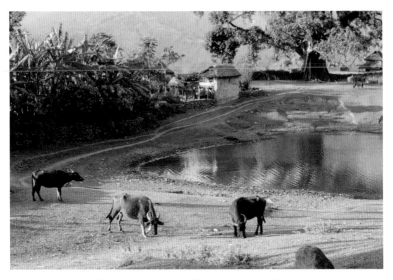

Water buffaloes in a quiet village, overlooked by a holy tree

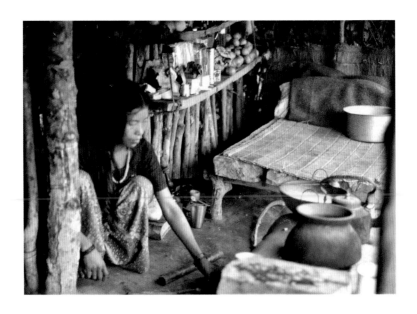

Tea houses emerge strategically along the main trails

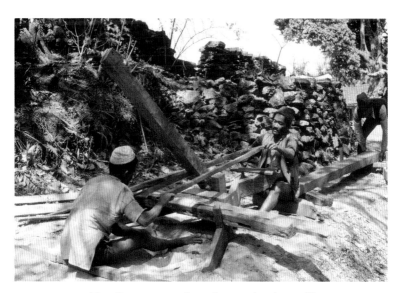

Nepali men operating a human lumber mill

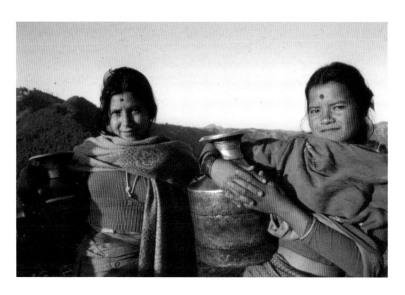

Women of all ages carry water for their households
Photo by Stephen Bezruchka

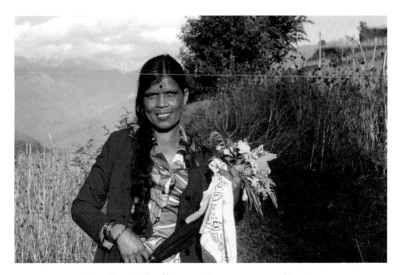

Sita Devi Khadka, vaccinator extraordinaire

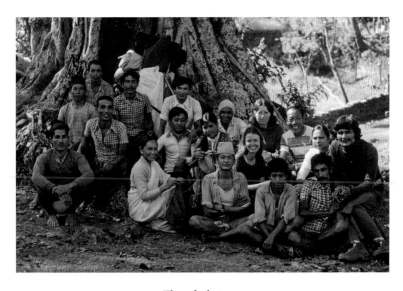

The whole team
Photo by Corinne Collins

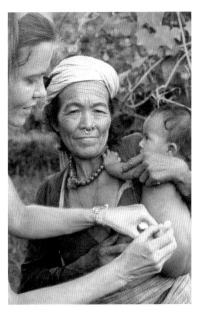

Our main job was immunizations—thousands of them
Photo by Jane Teas

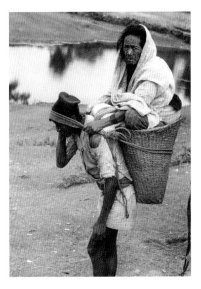

A village ambulance for transporting sick people to care

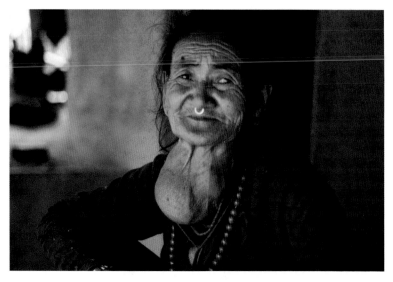

Some sought help for long-standing problems,
like this woman with a goiter

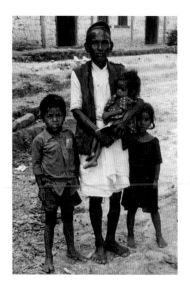

Life is difficult caring for
orphaned children

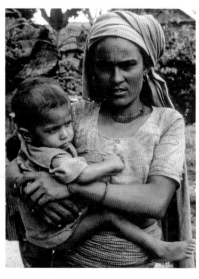

The classic signs of malnutrition
—thin and small for age,
thinning hair

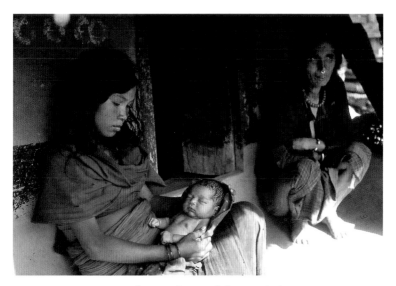

Sani, her mother, and the new baby

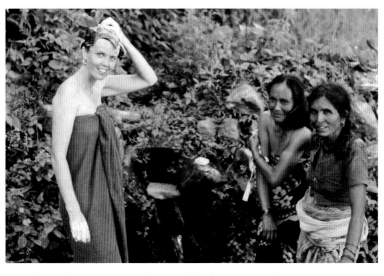

The author mastering the art of bathing at a public water source
Photo by Kate Jewell

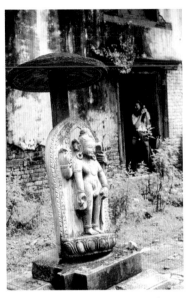

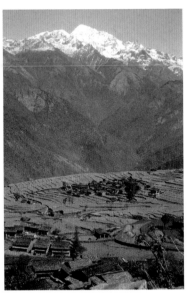

Exploring an abandoned
Rana police station
Photo by Jane Teas

The small village of Barpak
beneath Himalayan peaks

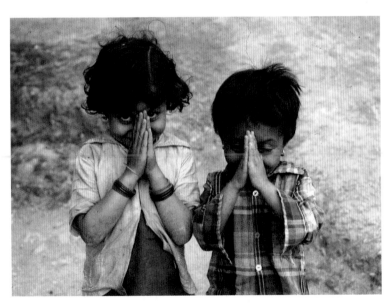

All children know how to "Namaste"—I honor the deity within you

Chapter 12
New Life

We bade a sad goodbye to Kate, who returned home to the States. Then, because of a particularly hard-to-reach set of villages in Aru Pokari, Corinne and I joined our teams together. I was ecstatic to have every evening with my good friend, which always involved gossiping and late-night chats in the tent we shared.

On our second morning, as the teams prepared to leave for the day's work, an older man came by the breakfast room. He looked at everyone quietly until one of the porters asked him to speak. Then he gave a worried look at Corinne and me and asked quietly if we could come and help his daughter. She was visiting the family home in a nearby village with her husband for a local festival and was in labor with her first baby.

"*Kati tem bhayo, Bau?*" I asked. *How long has it been, sir?*

"*Deraa din,* Memsaab," he answered.

A day and a half, pretty long even for a first baby. Corinne and I looked at each other with concern—but guarded concern. We had so much to do in this ward. The idea of delivering a baby was intriguing, but we wouldn't be able to complete the day's work if we left to do something else the first thing in the morning. It would be an exhausting day, with long treks to and from the immunization sites and the usual lines of sick people coming for *aushadi* (medicine).

"Let's ask him to wait a bit longer and see how it goes," I suggested to Corinne.

"Good idea."

So we sent the prospective grandfather home with reassurance, "You know, the first baby always takes longer, but come back if she doesn't deliver today."

That afternoon, all the teams arrived back at camp later than usual, and we gathered immediately for dinner.

"What's for dinner, Bhim Raj?" I joked.

"Ah, Mary Anne Didi, *dal bhat* today!" he replied with his usual grin. Bhim Raj was one of the few porters who seemed to get the Americans' attempts at humor. They were all a cheerful, laughing lot, but after a time I realized that humor had more cultural components than I had understood. I could always count on Bhim Raj to get the joke. Dinner was, of course, always *dal bhat*. Monotonous at first, I grew to anticipate that meal as if it were the blue plate special, appreciating the small variations in types of dal and spices. *Dal bhat* was what Nepali people ate, full stop. I often laughed at the impossible image of a Nepali child looking at her plate and whining, "But I don't LIKE *dal bhat*." It just didn't happen.

We were nearly finished eating when a local man stepped up to the doorway and asked if the Memsaabs could speak with a man from a nearby village. I went out to inquire and found the man who'd come that morning, his daughter still in labor. He seemed more concerned now, more anxious to have our help. There was a pleading in his voice that wasn't there this morning. He emphasized that he lived nearby and just wanted someone to come and see her, to see if there was anything we could do. I went back inside to consult with Corinne.

"Okay, Corinne, this is our chance. We've talked about how cool it would be to help with a home delivery—shall we do it?" I was ready for something to bring back my flagging sense of excitement about this life I was living. After nearly six months in the field, the sameness of each day's activities and the exhaustion that accompanied them sometimes had me yearning for a change—any change.

"I hope you know something about delivering babies, because I haven't been around one for a long time," Corinne replied. "But two days is a long time to be in labor. I wonder if we can do anything to help."

I'd been wondering the same thing. My six-week rotation in the maternity department during nursing school was all I knew about birthing, and that was ten years behind me. There would be, from this area, no possibility of referral to a hospital for a cesarean section, if that was needed. But after discussing the possibilities, we agreed that doing what we could with our limited knowledge was the only course to take. So, with a carry-bag containing an "OB kit" that included a few sterile instruments, a stethoscope, some antiseptic , sterile gloves, and (most importantly) a midwifery manual, we set out, following the old man out of camp and down the trail.

The sun was moving towards the horizon, but we estimated it would be light for at least another two hours, allowing us to get back to camp before dark. It had rained that morning, but most of the mud on the trail was dried up. We passed rice fields and farmsteads with goats, chickens, and children milling about the yards. The usual smell of cooking fires filled the air. The evening concert of cicadas was beginning as a gentle, almost imperceptible clicking whir. In some areas that sound would grow so intense I'd think I was hearing the machinery of a small factory, but this evening it was a peaceful lull.

"This won't exactly be close to camp, will it?" I muttered as we started down an especially steep part of the trail. I felt a familiar sense of annoyance rising in my chest. Why was everything so difficult here? Why couldn't the man just be honest about how far away he lived instead of misleading us into going there so late in the day? We'd just put in a full day's work, and I desperately wished for a good night's sleep.

Sure enough, we arrived at the house after nearly an hour, aware now that we wouldn't get back to camp that night. His home was just off the trail, closely surrounded by well-kept fields of millet and corn. We were ushered in to meet Maili, the young woman in labor, and the rest of her family. Though they were high-caste Brahmins, their few amenities and shabby clothing told us that they were quite poor, as many Brahmins were; even caste didn't protect against the poverty of the Nepali hills. Besides the father were the girl's husband, her mother, younger siblings, and grandmother, all very concerned and anxious about the difficult time Maili was having, and humbly grateful to us for coming to help.

After one look at Maili, my pique dissolved into compassion, and I resolved to make the trip worthwhile. A lovely young woman in her late teens with almond-shaped eyes, she was barely awake, face covered in sweat, exhausted beyond description after nearly two days of labor. She was the picture of misery.

This could be anybody, I thought to myself: my younger sister who had just given birth far away in America. Or my best friend, or anyone in a high-tech hospital at home. But all those women would have experts nearby, someone skilled who would know what to do, how to relieve the pain and make sure the result was a healthy baby and mother. Here there was just Corinne and me, and our best intentions. The realization slammed me in the face again: Life isn't easy, and it certainly isn't fair. Seeing Maili's condition, the responsibility weighed heavily.

Maili's husband sat beside her in the dark room on a straw mat, looking like any worried young father-to-be. Her pains were regular and fairly close together, but according to her mother, they hadn't changed in many hours. She moaned with each contraction, and her husband would reach over to massage her back and murmur something quietly in her ear. *Not like the typical Nepali man*, I mused, many of whom seemed to value their wives primarily for the work they did and children they bore. I wondered if they'd had a "love marriage" instead of an arranged one. The reassurance he was providing his young wife somehow comforted me as well.

"*Ke garne?*" asked the girl's mother, peering into our faces with a despairing look.

That ubiquitous Nepali phrase, indicating anything from puzzlement to—more often—resignation to the unseen forces of life, took on a new meaning. Right now it meant fear, anxiety. It filled every corner of the room.

We asked the husband to leave while we conducted an exam. Corinne and I each felt Maili's abdomen and listened with the stethoscope to find the heartbeat and determine if the baby was in the right position. We agreed that the head seemed to be down, in the right position, which was reassuring since a breech birth would have been much more worrisome. We could barely hear the baby's heart sounds, and they weren't exactly where we expected them to be loudest, but the rate was normal, an indicator that the baby was likely not in distress.

So why was her labor progressing so slowly?

Maili stirred, asking plaintively with half-open eyes if we could help her, but without a word of complaint for the agony she was enduring. "*Kasto dukkha, Maili. Abba bisek hunchha,*" I told her softly. *It hurts a lot, but soon it will be better.* I offered a silent prayer to whatever gods were watching that I was right.

We asked the family some questions, which revealed at least one reason for the long and unproductive labor: Maili's bag of waters hadn't broken yet. This would normally have occurred much earlier. The baby's head was being cushioned by fluid and wasn't effectively dilating her cervix, which an examination showed wasn't even halfway open, a miserably poor result after so much pain and effort.

Corinne and I looked at each other intently. "What do you think?" she asked. We realized at the same time that there was something we could do: use an instrument to rupture the bag of waters. It was a simple medical procedure, but one that neither of us had done before.

To carry out this medical procedure would be to cross the line between what was expected of us as nurses and what we believed was needed. How many times had we heard the mantra from our Foundation boss that our job was not to "treat the natives," but to provide immunizations and talk about health. Corinne and I had agreed how unfair and also ineffective that approach was. The villagers understandably believed that we were coming to help with their problems—the problems that they lived with, day after day. Why would they cooperate with strangers who only wanted to stick needles in their children to prevent some disease they barely knew existed?

The procedure we were contemplating, though simple technically, was risky for several reasons: It might not be effective; it might lead to complications such as infection; and, even more frightening, if it wasn't effective and there were serious remaining problems with the delivery, we could be blamed. I'd heard stories of Nepali doctors in rural districts who refused to perform critical procedures because if they failed and the patient died, family members would retaliate. Sometimes the result was physical violence towards the doctor—a kind of vigilante malpractice suit.

We contemplated our options and pored over the midwifery manual.

"Should we do it?" asked Corinne, her eyes wide with both uncertainty and a hint of anticipation.

Intervening meant assuming more responsibility for this young woman than we'd planned when we set out: a commitment to see her through her delivery, however long it took. Things could go wrong, really wrong. Before coming to Nepal I'd worked in a post-earthquake relief camp in Guatemala. I remembered the horror of a delivery attended by the camp doctor that went bad, resulting in a dead baby and very traumatized mother. Could we take that chance?

We discussed our choices. Maili might do just fine without us, or she could stay in this condition another day or two. There was no need to put into words the other possible outcomes.

Maili gave another moan. Corinne shrugged and shook her head slowly. "We can't just leave her here, can we?" she asked brightly. "We do have a sterile ring forceps."

The decision was made.

Five minutes later we'd assembled our equipment, asked the family to step outside, and carried out the procedure, painstakingly following each step described in the midwifery manual. A gush of fluid rewarded our efforts, and we settled back to see what happened next. Would labor speed up? Had we done the right thing? Was it enough?

Soon, Maili's labor seemed to progress more effectively, but by that time it was 11:00 p.m. and a soft rain had begun to patter on the thatched rooftop. We couldn't return to camp now, so Corinne and I prepared to camp on the covered veranda of the family's house. The light of a kerosene lantern softened the rounded red-brown contours of our sleeping area. All the usual voices and other sounds of night-time activity were gone now, except for the cicadas and the occasional yelp of a neighborhood dog. The aroma of cooking fires had wafted away on the cool night air.

We decided to take turns monitoring Maili's progress. I took the first shift, seating myself against the wall near her. Maili would drop off to sleep every three to four minutes between contractions, awaken to moan softly, and then doze again, her husband still beside her. My mind drifted to night shifts I'd spent as a student in the maternity ward, marveling that though the settings couldn't have been more different, they were alike in those human dimensions: anticipation of new life dulled by the pain of bringing it forth.

A maze of conflicts wove in and out around me. The intense concern from all Maili's family, and their inability to do anything to help her except, as a last resort, call on these foreign strangers. Our own concern for Maili, the timeless kinship of women with other laboring women, despite massive differences in our lives. The midwifery manual, helpful as it was, pitted us against the centuries old birthing traditions. And mostly, Maili's pain, erasing all reality for her except each successive contraction, even the hope for what would come.

"Aaahh—what's biting me out here?" came a wail from Corinne. "Every time I drift off to sleep, I wake up with some little critter attacking me. It's driving me nuts!"

I went out to the veranda to investigate and found a frantic Corinne. "Look at this!" My flashlight, dim as it was with a half-used battery, revealed dozens of tiny bites on her back, her legs, her arms.

Corinne and I had come to terms with the ever-present insect pests in Nepal: deep swarms of flies wherever we went during the day and pesky mosquitoes lurking in the tent at night. The worst so far had been the fleas, which had an affinity for bodily sites covered most tightly with clothing. The itching at night was so intense that for a time we tried wearing doggie flea collars around our waists. But these bites were something new, which later we learned were probably bedbugs that infested the sleeping porch.

When my turn came to sleep, I had the same problem. At ten- or fifteen-minute intervals, I'd be startled awake by tiny pinching bites. I'd emit a moan, a sigh, and try to find a corner away from the little devils. *Oh please, let this night be over soon,* I thought, over and over. We all spent a miserable night—though Maili's piteous moans reminded us how very comfortable we were in comparison with her endless pain.

Finally, dawn began to brighten the sky and glorious fountains of birdsong filled the air. Corinne stirred, groaned, and whispered apologetically, "I really have to get back to camp and away from these

bugs! I don't think I've slept more than half an hour all night. Sorry
to leave you here, but we have a lot to do today and somebody's got to
get the team moving. I'd better go."

I agreed that we weren't both needed, and I'd stick around. Looking
disheveled and miserable, Corinne set out on the trail toward camp.

Now it was up to me. A curious thought struck me: *Why am I not
more worried?* I was outside the limits of my professional skills; what
was now a labor of over two days qualified as an obstetric complication by any standard medical definition, and I clearly wasn't trained
or experienced to handle it. But something about the setting gave me
the sense, foolish as it was, that whatever happened was supposed to
happen.

Have I been in Nepal too long? I wondered. *Ke garne*, accept the
inevitable, realize the limitations of mere humans to affect the course
of events. It was how so many Nepali villagers coped with a lifetime
onslaught of problems beyond their control—but me? I was from
the tradition of dealing with challenges, solving problems, fighting
injustice. What was happening to me?

I turned my attention back to Maili, whose pains were more
intense now, closer together. She cried out with each pain, rather
than emitting the low moans of the night. I took another short rest
on the veranda. Then at 7:30 sharp, her mother beckoned: The baby
is coming. As I moved back into position, she and the grandmother
crouched behind me, ready to let me produce whatever magic I could
conjure up. Indeed, the top of the baby's head was barely visible now
with each contraction, the last stage before birth. I murmured a few
words of encouragement to Maili, "You're doing so well, the baby will
be coming soon," praying that it would finally be true.

The mother-to-be lay on the same straw mat where she'd been
throughout her labor. I realized with annoyance that we hadn't
packed a clean surface to use for the delivery, so there could be no
semblance of sterility. But I was given a clean cloth, and I spread it on

the mat beneath the laboring woman. The room was shadowy, with just the door and one small window to let in the hopeful rays of the morning sun. Propping up my ever-present flashlight into a position to give me some view of what was happening, I waited. Maili tried to push, but she was so exhausted that each push seemed less and less effective. Many minutes passed—how many, fifteen? twenty?—with no further progress.

I took deep breaths again, imagining the deliveries I'd witnessed at Mayo Clinic during my training. I remembered the frequent practice of episiotomy, a small cut in the vaginal opening. Should I do that? How much longer can she keep this up? What else was there to do? Corinne wasn't around to consult, nor was anyone else. Like so many medical procedures, the use of episiotomy was found years later to be rarely needed and often dangerous, but at the time it was standard practice for many physicians. I decided to proceed.

Carefully drawing a pair of sterile scissors out of the package, I winced at the prospect of using them. Maili's pains were so intense that she likely wouldn't feel the cut, but I squirmed at the thought of snipping into the living tissue of another human being, something I'd never done before. There was no possibility of anesthesia, or sutures afterwards. Though I expected that a small cut would heal on its own better than a larger tear, my choices still seemed equally bad. Finally, I decided I couldn't watch Maili slip more deeply into her state of total exhaustion. She needed help, and I was it.

I made the cut, just as I remembered seeing it done a lifetime ago in sterile delivery rooms.

Then with the next contraction, like a small explosion, with one smooth thrust a full-size baby boy slithered into my hands. I held his slippery body carefully, awed, and inhaled that unique musky scent of amniotic fluid that accompanies every new human being's entrance into the world. He took some tiny breaths and then let out a strong, indignant cry. His little head was grotesquely elongated from the many hours in labor, but he was healthy, he was pink, he was alive!

Maili and her mother watched him look around at his new surroundings, and smiled with relief and joy. Realizing how strong the "son preference" was in Nepal, I knew it was auspicious for the family that this was a boy, making all the pain and effort fully worthwhile. A girl would also have been wonderful, but for them, not as wonderful. I rejoiced with them, as Maili's grandmother stepped outside to spread the news of the birth.

I started to tie the umbilical cord, but my effort was abruptly stopped with a cry of "*Pardaina!*"—*No, we can't do that*—indicating I had to wait for the placenta to be delivered. She gave no reason, and I guessed that this was one of those long-standing practices that women in this culture "just did." Much later the standard medical practice of immediate cord-cutting was rejected, when it was found that waiting until maximum amounts of blood flowed to the baby would help prevent anemia. But knowing of no harm in a delay, I sat back to await this important final stage of the delivery. I couldn't relax yet, but I was smiling proudly in my mind, preparing to tell the tale back at camp.

Various family members drifted in to look at the baby, worry about the elongation of his head, and smile at me. I reassured everyone that his skull would go back to a normal shape after a few weeks. Maili's mother repeated the story of our sleepless night, the insect bites, and our kindness to Maili to everyone who came by. She smiled with gratitude, and I understood that her gracious manner meant "thank you," even though there is no word or phrase for that specific sentiment in the Nepali language. Children appeared at the window, peeked in, and left. Except for the long duration, it was a classic home birth, with family support in a familiar environment (however, as in most traditional settings, the men were absent when the real action started). The grandmother started a fire in the corner for the morning meal.

Finally, as I was beginning to worry that Maili was having another problem, the placenta emerged intact. A critical moment, since many of the deaths from hemorrhage or infection after a delivery occur when some of the placenta is left behind. I made sure her bleeding was minimal, and the entire party went outside for the cord cutting.

Maili's mother carried the baby into the bright morning, attached placenta and all. I crouched down beside them in the warm sunlight. With two quick ties and one cut of the scissors later—intently observed by the bevy of family members—my work was done. The grandmother came out to bathe the baby with what must have felt like ice water on his velvety skin. To prevent an infection after such a long labor—not to mention our interventions—I gave the family a package of antibiotics to give Maili over the next week.

I suddenly realized that a thin veil of anxiety, a pall that I had nearly stopped noticing, had left me. For whatever reason—our simple actions, fate, the gods, or dumb luck—things had turned out fine. Good mother, good baby. All the images of bad outcomes, the tragedies that could have happened, left my mind as quickly as they'd arrived. I'd done my best and it was enough—at least this time.

I looked around to say goodbye to Maili and noted that she'd already been isolated with her baby, away from the rest of the family, settled into a small cubicle lined with straw mats on the veranda. In the Nepali culture, as in many others, childbirth is considered a highly polluting process. The mother has to have a period of ritual purification after the delivery, eating special foods, isolated from others. Although the practice had seemed cruel (and definitely strange) when I first learned about it, over time it seemed reasonable and practical. Maili needed time to rest, to regain her strength, and the baby needed to be protected from exposure to infections until his immune system was more developed. Like so many of the customs that initially seemed pointless, there was some logic to this Nepali version of maternity leave.

Neighbors began drifting by to get the news, and morning in the village began as it always had: with men discussing the day's work ahead, women at the cooking fires, children giggling and sneaking peeks at the foreign woman in their midst, while chickens scratched out their morning meals.

It was one of those perfect Nepali mornings that felt more like home than any other place I'd lived since leaving my family's Montana ranch. This wasn't an uncomplicated world, but one where everyone had a place, no one was superfluous, and the outside world didn't matter a lot. Something about this experience could have happened in the little rural area where I grew up, I realized. In a wave of homesickness, I wished that my parents were near; both my mother and father would truly appreciate the joy of these moments. I'd have to make do with writing it down in my weekly letter home.

I said my goodbyes and started up the trail back to camp. Clearly the village grapevine had preceded me, because soon the queries began from houses I passed:

"Chhora ki chhori?" Boy or girl?

"Chhora ho!" I responded with an excited smile. *It's a boy!*

Eventually I moved along the trail in silence, and the elation of a happy outcome gave way to second thoughts. The image of that baby emerging at the final moment of birth kept flashing into my mind. Something about it was odd. What was it?

Then, like a textbook picture, there it was: The baby came out face up, not face down as they most commonly do. I jerked to a stop and, looking for a place to pull together my thoughts, sat down on a large boulder. Aii! No wonder it took so long. Maili had had a posterior presentation, which nearly always means a more difficult birth. We should have figured it out sooner, when we heard the baby's heartbeat in such an odd place, and tried some maneuvers to help the baby move into better position. Damn! The molding of the head wasn't just because of the long labor—his position had added to it. It was obvious, looking back. So much for my great expertise.

I sighed, and reminded myself that, despite our uncertainty, we did the right thing to get the labor moving, and it ended well. But if I needed convincing, the harsh reality of this one experience showed me how desperately pregnant women—all pregnant women—need someone with skills to turn to when childbearing becomes a nightmare of unending pain and risk.

The night had been a jolting contrast from my work in the US. As a hospital nurse and even as a nurse practitioner, there were clear limits to what I was allowed to do. For the most part they involved compliantly following protocols and doctors' orders, doing as I was instructed. I always did that well, an obedient and well-behaved woman. But something was happening to me in these Nepali hills: Pure necessity had shown me who else I could be—and I liked it.

Chapter 13
Visitors

"So you really do this every day, no matter what the weather?" asked Jane. I had just slipped in my flip-flops on a wet section of the trail, smearing red mud all over the seat of my denim skirt. Muddy hands, muddy feet, muddy clothes, the joy of trekking during the rainy season. I sighed.

"Yeah, afraid so. Otherwise we'd have to quit for several months, and that wouldn't have made any sense. It's definitely a bit . . . inconvenient at times," I admitted. "Anyway, the monsoon is pretty much over now, so it'll get easier."

I'd met Jane on a previous trip to Kathmandu. Having just finished her doctoral degree studying primate behavior at the Kathmandu temples, she was eager to see the rural areas and agreed to join me for a few days of work. It was delightful to have someone from my own culture to share the long days in the field. She spoke some Nepali, and although she was almost as tall as I was, her black hair helped her to blend in with the local women more easily than I did.

After a long downhill trek, we found the day's immunization site near the center of a small village. We set up shop, and the women began trickling in with their frightened-looking kids. I gave the injections, and Jane restrained the children when needed. Then she had the gratifying job of providing a piece of hard candy to the little ones when their ordeal was over. I was, as usual, approached by villagers seeking help for a cough, a pain, or a sore somewhere—which I often couldn't provide.

Towards the end of the day, as we began packing up to leave, a small family group approached us. The mother and two small children hugging close to her skirts looked healthy and remarkably clean, given all the mud we were living in. But the child in her arms was a desolate-looking, whiny baby with the old man skin-and-bones look of marasmus, the most serious level of malnutrition.

The mother approached with a plaintive look, saying the child was sick and asking if I had medicine for her. She sat down with me on a nearby bench, Jane standing behind us. The sight of this pathetic waif, covered only by a threadbare cloth, stopped my breath for a moment. Her face was a picture of misery, her little limbs showed every detail of the bones that pushed out against thin, flaky skin.

"How old is your baby?" I asked the mother, trying to sound helpful and professional, and struggling not to show the horror I felt. I'd seen malnourished children, but none as skeletal as this one.

"*Tin barsa laagyo,*" she replied. *Almost three.* I suppressed a gasp and noted a look of concern in Jane's eyes. The little girl, who looked less than half that age, let out a faint moan and moved restlessly in her mother's arms.

I gave a cursory exam and asked about the course of the child's symptoms, the family circumstances, and what had been done to date. The story she told was a variant of one I'd heard many times already for malnourished children. She had been doing okay until she was about a year old, when a younger brother was born, displacing her from the breast. After that she didn't gain weight and stopped eating, getting steadily thinner. They hadn't been to a medical clinic, but instead took her to a traditional healer or *jhakri*.

"And what did the *jhakri* do?" I asked. "Did it help?"

The mother described a procedure called *putlaa garne*: The *jhakri* went over the child's body with his mouth, biting and searching for the source of the disease. He came out with something like a piece of sinew in his mouth, which he said was causing the problem and that his removing it should cure the child.

Clearly the procedure hadn't helped. What could I tell her? The chance of recovery for a child this badly malnourished was very slim, and I didn't want to give false hope to the mother, who obviously was concerned and caring. If I gave advice for what to do and it failed, as it almost certainly would, she would bear added guilt for the little girl's death.

Choosing the middle ground, I explained that the only real answer for this problem was food, describing how to prepare the simple protein-calorie mix recommended for weaning children. But I added that it might be too late for that to work.

"*Ekdum gaaro chha, hoina?*" I said, with a frown of sympathy. *It's very hard, isn't it?*

"*Gaaro,*" she agreed, with a look of defeat, as if this was the verdict she expected. She rose, gathered the other children, gave a nod of thanks, and walked away.

Jane and I didn't speak for a while after the family left. Finally I said, "That was an extreme case, but I see this kind of problem quite a bit. It's discouraging. These kids need more than our immunizations. They're more likely to die of malnutrition or diarrhea or pneumonia or measles than anything we can immunize against."

Jane just shook her head. "Pretty sad, eh?" she said softly.

We packed up the rest of our supplies in preparation for the two-hour (uphill, of course) trek back to camp. As we started out, a hesitant male voice came from behind me.

"Memsaab, namaste," I heard. Turning around, I saw that it was the husband of Maili, the woman whose baby I'd delivered the previous week. He smiled happily as I greeted him.

"Namaste, Daai. *Kasto chha?*" I asked.

"*Sabbai raamro,* Memsaab," he answered. *Everything's fine.* We continued with a short conversation about how the baby was eating, and how Maili was feeling. All indeed seemed well.

I felt a small flame of satisfaction coming from somewhere deep inside. I'd actually done something worthwhile, I mused. This mom and her healthy baby were evidence that I could be useful. A rare validation, since I almost never had follow-up information on those I took care of.

But this was just a single case. As my time in Gorkha had worn on, week after exhausting week, my feeling grew that the results of all my efforts weren't worth the energy expended. This visit from Jane was a chance to talk out all my doubts and uncertainty, feelings I didn't think I should share with my teammates.

We slogged back to camp, taking our time as the late afternoon air began to cool. I glimpsed the welcome sight of our tents when one of the porters jogged up to us, looking excited. "They've been waiting for you, Memsaab," he said and beckoned us to follow him. *Oh, right.* I had been told that the school near where we were camped was having a program, and we were to be the honored guests.

"Sorry, Jane, I forgot about this," I said with a slight grimace. She smiled and gave a Nepali nod.

Makeshift curtains had been strung between two trees in front of the village meeting house to enclose the stage. We were seated in the place of honor—not just the best, they were in fact the only seats in the house: a couple of rickety chairs close to the front. The rest of the crowd sat on mats on the ground, or milled around at the back.

Time passed—ten minutes, fifteen minutes—and the crowd of spectators grew. *Well, clearly they weren't waiting too long for us,* I thought. Finally, the sounds of drumming and a wavering girl's voice singing a popular Nepali song wafted out, just as the curtains were being dragged apart slowly by two small sets of hands. The crowd cheered and clapped at the sight of a group of middle school–aged children standing in one straight line who had joined in singing the opening song.

I had been curious to see how a small Nepali school event would compare to the Christmas programs at my childhood one-room school in rural Montana. Those were uniquely memorable occasions in my childhood. The whole community came, even the old bachelor brothers who lived down the road from us. My first performance there was at the age of five, reciting "Twas the Night Before Christmas" in its entirety (an experience that made me wary of public speaking ever after, even though my parents told me it went without a hitch). There was a comforting familiarity about it all. When the program was over, the audience clapped and shouted their approval.

Jane and I rose, making our namastes to the teachers. We quickly took the evening meal, said final good nights to the team, and crawled into the tent.

"So this is what it's like for you," commented Jane, as we settled into our sleeping bags. "Much more interesting and real than Kathmandu, but harder too. At least it would be difficult for me."

The frustrations and fatigue of the past few months suddenly rose up in my chest like an evil spirit clamoring to get out. *Yes! Difficult!*

"Really, I'm more exhausted after six months than I've ever been in my life," I sighed. "I'm supposed to be here for another full year, and I don't know if I can make it that long. I feel like such a wimp, but right now I'm depressed at the thought of it."

What a relief. I had let myself say it out loud, and it sounded even truer than when it was cloistered in my mind. *Something about this work is hard. Maybe too hard for me.* The words were both liberating and frightening.

I waited for Jane's response. She had been given a glimpse of my world, and I was anxious to hear what she made of it.

"Well, I guess I would probably feel the same way," offered Jane. "You're being asked to bring twentieth-century technology to people who are still living in the sixteenth century." She hesitated, then added, "You're constantly on the go, so you don't have a chance to get to know the people in the villages you're supposed to be helping. There's so much to understand about their lives, but you never get to stop working and spend that kind of time with them."

I thought for a moment about Jane's comment, which brought an anthropologist's view to the work I was doing. I hadn't envisioned our constant activity and travel in those terms, but her words rang true. Not only did I rarely have follow-up on my work, I also had very little opportunity to interact with the people I met after the children's shots were given, the advice provided, and medicine passed out.

"It's true. There are so many things that make it hard, and I just . . ." My voice trailed off as I tried to imagine the options that were open to me. "I don't know how I can quit, after only six months," I sighed. "Maybe if I had a good long break it would help. I'll have to think about that when I get back to Kathmandu."

We said our good nights and I soon heard the sound of Jane's slow, even breathing. I lay awake for a while longer, trying without success to imagine a satisfactory path ahead. Where could I go from here?

I couldn't deny how much I was learning, as the weeks went by. This job was burning into my brain vivid images of the living conditions that were probably much the same as those of the many other poor countries of the world. A "subsistence economy" had just been a vague technical term before I saw it as a day-to-day reality. Now it meant struggling to have what most consider a normal life: enough food, respectable clothing, medical care if they or their children needed it, and even a few moments of leisure now and then. But there was also beauty in their lives, particularly a real sense of community that was being lost with every successive generation in the world I'd come from. I knew that those vaguely seen "others" living in countries of the South, who were only in the news when they suffered droughts, floods, or famines, would never again be a kind of generality to me. Being with them every day, as privileged as I was, I felt a growing sense of solidarity, particularly with women and the complicated lives they lived.

The next morning, Jane and I were both cheerful as we loaded up our daypacks under a sunny, post-monsoon sky. We were headed to Kathmandu, and the trek back to the highway would be a long one. Dhawa, at the edge of Gorkha district and the shortest route to where the Foundation car was scheduled to pick us up, would take over twelve hours. Out of respect for the unknown trails ahead, I traded my usual flip-flops for a deteriorating pair of well-worn tennis shoes.

The long trail back to the highway began as expected: an endless series of ups and downs, rarely level except when we followed the river. Jane and I chatted intermittently. As the hours passed, my mind drifted to imagining what I would do during my four days in Kathmandu.

Then the rocky trail we were following turned into a cobbled pathway, half-covered with dirt and vegetation. Very soon we saw an unexpected sight off to the right: In the middle of the dense forest, otherwise broken only by the path, rose an ancient-looking stone wall. Growing closer, I saw it obscured a larger two-story brick building, partially covered in crumbling plaster. The building consisted of one large room, with a long hallway off to the left that led into many smaller rooms. The doors and windows were framed with ornately carved wood in the style of the older Kathmandu buildings. In front was a courtyard, with a small temple in the center and nearby a beautifully intact statue of one of the Hindu gods listing at an awkward angle. Masses of weeds, vines, and pieces of other broken statues strewn about indicated there had been no attempt for many years to maintain what must have once been a beautiful complex.

I was excited. Something mysterious and unexpected! We wandered in and out of the rooms, trying to understand what history these abandoned ruins might convey.

"What on earth is it?" Jane asked. "What an amazing thing to find out here, near no villages at all."

I asked the porter what he made of the structures, and he replied matter-of-factly that it was a police station, from the Rana era.

That made sense. The Rana dynasty, a powerful, high-caste family that had ruled Nepal for over a century, spent inordinate resources on exerting their power over the population. Police stations based in rural areas were used to monitor and maintain order of the often rebellious citizens. The fall of that dynasty in 1951 explained why this outpost had been abandoned.

Looking over the ruins and their lost beauty, I wondered how many more of these relics were scattered about the country, remnants of this fascinating and violent political drama from Nepal's history. The century-long Rana rule had begun with a massacre in 1848 that was laced with high intrigue, royal family rivalries, and the assassination of a sitting prime minister (said to have been the queen's lover). After the slaughter of dozens of the leading Nepali nobles and their followers, the Rana victor appointed himself prime minister and sent the king and queen into exile. The royal prince was placed under house arrest, as were his descendants for the next hundred years.

Though the Rana rule was eventually overthrown, I could not have imagined that over twenty years after my time in Gorkha, in 2001, another royal family massacre at the Royal Palace in Kathmandu would eventually lead to a final end of the monarchy.

"So this is how the Ranas were able to stay in power for a hundred years," I commented to Jane. "Their police were everywhere. Pretty remarkable."

"Their palaces in Kathmandu are impressive, too, in a sick kind of way," she replied. "How much of the way these village people live now is because of the Ranas? There wasn't much effort to build up the rural areas."

As we were snapping pictures, I suddenly noticed that the afternoon sun was well on its downward drift toward the horizon. It was a beautiful, cloudless day, but I knew that when night fell it came very quickly.

"Hey, we'd better get moving," I called out to Jane. "We're still quite a long way from the road." We loaded up our daypacks and set out again, more hurried than before.

We had paid a price for the historical detour. After a few hours, the sun set over the distant hills and dusk turned to darkness. I asked the porter how much farther it would be to our destination.

"*Dui-tin ganta,* Memsaab," he replied. *Two or three hours.* There was no thought of stopping now.

I was uncertain at first about venturing down what had become a steeper path, flanked by low bushes on one side and a rock face on the other. My flashlight was out of reach, at the bottom of the porter's pack, and anyway the cheap batteries would only last for an hour or so. But soon the moon rose, and though I had no idea of what lay outside the edges of the narrow trail, we could see well enough to continue cautiously. For two more hours we descended the mostly downhill path under the lunar glow, only once getting briefly off the main route.

Just as I was wondering if we were going to be walking all night, the trail flattened out and we came to a clearing near a small home. Our porter shouted out a greeting to the householders, and eventually an older man came hobbling out, clearly roused from sleep. He told us that we were not far from the highway, and we were welcome to stop there for the night. Jane and I looked at each other and gave deep sighs of relief.

As we unpacked our gear, a small contingent of family members—a much younger wife and several children of various ages—gathered around. They peered at us intently as we put up the tent, and then when we retreated into it, disappeared back into the house.

"Always the main show," I commented to Jane as we settled for the night. By now she understood my annoyance with the constant observation that was my reality in Gorkha.

Early the next morning as we broke camp and prepared to leave, I glanced back at where we'd come from the previous evening and was startled by what I saw.

"Check that out, Jane," I commented. "I'm glad we didn't know that's where we were last night." She turned back to look. The trail we had traversed in the dark stretched back and up a circuitous-looking route for as far as I could see. Though most of it was bordered by low shrubbery, there were abrupt, steep drops in many places from the trail edge. It was unnerving to see how close we were to disaster had one of us slipped off in the darkness.

Another surprise awaited us. The highway was on the opposite side of the nearby river, which could be crossed in only two ways. One was to hike another hour or so upstream to a small bridge and then back again. The other was to do what the locals did, cross the river in an open wooden box, about two feet by three feet in size, suspended by flimsy looking ropes from a heavy metal cable. The operator of the *tuin*, as it was called, perched on the side of the cage and took passengers or cargo across the river in the box by pulling it by hand to the other side.

"*Yeseri janne?*" asked the porter. *Are we going on this?*

Jane and I looked at each other and the tumultuous gray river rushing below us. The cable ran from steep banks on both sides of the water. An image of what would happen if for any reason the system failed and it dropped into the water far below gave me a sudden spasm in my gut. *Very unlikely, of course*, I assured myself. This has probably been in use for ages. But still . . . everyone had heard tragic stories of accidents on Nepal's shaky transportation systems.

I gave a faked cheerful grin at Jane. "Guess we should, eh?" I said, trying to sound confident. The alternative of another couple of hours walking back and forth to the closest bridge was not appealing.

She answered back with a nod and a small smile. Okay, another adventure.

I paid the operator his small fee. Jane stepped into the box and sat up against one side, and I followed, squeezing myself in opposite her. The little box felt insubstantial, unstable. The *tuin* operator, a thin, ragged man with burly forearms, jumped onto the edge of the box after us and quickly pushed off from the bank. My stomach lurched at the first rapid surge, swooping downward toward the center of the river, reminding me of those first few moments of a carnival ride. I gripped the wooden slats and closed my eyes. Pitching forward, we descended even closer to the river and its soft roar. Then we slowed, seeming to hesitate at the lowest point between the two banks. I opened my eyes to narrow slits and looked down, trying to calm my anxious thoughts . . . *I wonder what's wrong. Why aren't we going the rest of the way?* Then our *tuin* operator went to work, slowly pulling us hand-over-hand to the other side. With one last upward swing we halted abruptly on the other high bank.

Jumping out, I allowed myself a deep breath and a smile. Our belongings followed with the porter. From the landing it was a brief walk to the road, and then a welcome sight: The bright yellow Foundation jeep was waiting just off the highway. Gopal, who was driving, pulled up beside us, smiling when I complimented him on his perfect timing. We paid the porter, threw our bags into the car, and sat back to be transported, effortlessly, luxuriously, to Kathmandu.

As much as I wanted to shut out everything except the lull of the highway and plans for my next few days of city life, discussions with Jane kept popping back into my mind. *Yes, this job was hard, and no, not because I was a wimp. Another year, another year,* was the dreaded thought that I couldn't suppress. How much longer could I stay in Gorkha, spending endless hours on the trail, going to new villages with the same old problems, and feeling oppressed by a layer of gloom too much of the time?

Jane had helped me understand that is was not just the physical challenge that oppressed me; I was getting used to that, though still exhausted most evenings. A sense of continuity, of depth in my daily contacts with the village people was lacking.

Under that sadness was something else: a dark undercurrent of loneliness. I could see that as the months went on, I was mourning less for the marriage I'd left behind. But rather than lifting a burden, it left a void that wasn't even close to being filled. Much as I was growing to love Sita and the others on my team, their experience of the world was light-years away from mine. I was incredibly fortunate to have Corinne as a friend and confidant, but she also had the satisfying diversion of a boyfriend in Kathmandu. I felt oddly alone in this adventure.

Within three hours, we were at the outskirts of Kathmandu, where I would be immersed back in the pleasures of city life. Food choices, movies at the Embassy, shopping for trinkets in the bazaar, a pillow-soft bed where I could sprawl out. Indoor plumbing, a steaming shower.

But I'd come back to Kathmandu because a staff member from our Foundation, Fred, was in town from his New York office. The very next morning the entire expatriate staff met with him for a briefing on the state of the organization, his observations of our efforts, and a general discussion about the months ahead.

"Great to see you all, and meet a few of you I haven't met before," Fred began, smiling an official welcome. Tall, blond, and athletic looking, he spoke with a booming voice and the tone of someone who was accustomed to giving pro forma speeches.

After commenting on the great work we were doing, he launched into a series of issues he wanted to discuss. Uniforms: Until now, we all wore whatever clothing was most comfortable, but he had brought with him a box of custom-ordered shirts with logos in Foundation colors that he wanted us to wear when in the field. He seemed particularly concerned that no one was tempted to "go native," meaning dressing like local women. Photos: Fundraising depended on his having good pictures of us at work, particularly ones that showed the Foundation logo on equipment or clothing. Medicines: He had brought a box of drugs and other supplies that he wanted to be sure were available to us in case needed by staff (but not, he added, for others). Finally, he proudly displayed a few expensive-looking "gifts" for us, including a charming wicker picnic basket with plastic plates and cutlery.

Towards the end of the "discussion," which was almost entirely Fred talking to us, I felt a growing annoyance. He was a direct, candid communicator, which I appreciated. But medicines, just for us, not for the sick people we saw in the villages? Expensive shirts to advertise the Foundation's presence in villages? A picnic set, when every day was by definition a "picnic"? The meeting ended without any real dialogue with staff.

Over the next few days, I asked about people's reactions to the comments from our headquarters rep and found that those who knew him already were unsurprised and unconcerned. It struck me as odd that he didn't plan to make a trip to see our field activities, though other key staff members from New York made that a key part of their visits. After our meeting, Fred was occupied with meeting local dignitaries, and we interacted with him only informally. Then the day before Corinne and I were scheduled to return to Gorkha, we sat with him and other staff over lunch in our Chabahil residence. Fred launched forth in a professorial tone.

"So, I'd love to hear more about how things are going in the field," he opened. "You should know I've told Corinne that you're going to have to find a way to get more kids vaccinated—70 percent just doesn't cut it. So you'll have to work harder, or better, and aim for at least 80 percent everywhere. Ideas about how you can do that?"

Work harder? I thought, stung by the comment. He's got to be kidding. And then the dam burst: Six months of frustration and angst spewed forth.

"Do you really mean that?" I asked, feeling heat rising in my cheeks. "Work harder? Do you know what it's like out there? We're going twelve hours every day as it is. It's really exhausting, and I for one don't see any way we can work much harder."

There was a moment of silence. Fred looked around at the rest of the small group.

"Well, Mary Anne, I'm very sorry to hear that," he said slowly, and I waited for the punch line that was clearly coming. "I wonder if you appreciate the real privilege you have in doing this work. I can promise you there are many others who would happily step into your shoes. Anyone who doesn't like this work shouldn't be here. They should probably just go home," he thundered.

The last comment put me over the edge I'd been teetering on.

"Sir, I just might have to do that," I answered his challenge, shaking my head sadly, stood up abruptly, and left the room.

As I stalked off into the corridor and then outside to go somewhere—anywhere—on my bicycle, I had an odd feeling of triumph mixed with disbelief. Was that me? I was not the "just tell them off, say what you think" kind of person. But I'd done just that.

It was time to face the complicated set of feelings I had for this job, this life. In the end, it seemed to point in one direction: I couldn't stay on for another year.

Chapter 14
Hard Choices

What a relief! Getting back to Gorkha, away from the furious activity of Kathmandu, the crowds and the noise and diesel smells of buses and trucks, felt like breaking out of prison. I decided to wait a few weeks before figuring when to submit my resignation. I was mostly just putting off the decision, but was still convinced it had to happen.

On the trek together back to Gorkha village, Corinne and I indulged in *gaf garne*, loosely translated as gossiping, which whiled away some of the ten-hour trip. Even the dreaded climb up Cheppetar Hill was less arduous than I remembered. Maybe it was the company, or because I could now see an end to the eternal trails, or maybe I was getting in better shape. Most likely all three.

"Doesn't it seem odd that Fred isn't coming to Gorkha to see our actual work?" I remarked as we sat at our first teahouse stop, sipping the sweet, hot brew. "There's not that much happening in Kathmandu. But it's a lot of work to get out here," I said, rolling my eyes. "Too much work for him, I guess." I still rankled at his implication that we weren't working hard enough in the field. However, my annoyance turned to gratitude when, a year later, the Foundation president gave me a sparkling reference for my application for the Master of Public Health degree at Johns Hopkins University. That program launched the rest of my career in public health.

"Listen, we know what we're doing, even if he doesn't," asserted Corinne. She was ever loyal to her team, somehow maintaining a calm reaction to the previous day's pronouncements while loyally supporting our efforts.

We arrived at the Gorkha house in plenty of time for a cold beer, a hot supper, and a good night's sleep. The next morning, the two teams headed back to our separate sites.

The trek to our next *panchayat*, Borlang, was relatively cool after a night of heavy rain. We passed by rice paddies that had turned a Day-Glo chartreuse, adding a colorful new dimension to the terraced hillsides. The porters and vaccinators chattered and bantered as we made our way along the trail, giving the sense that we were out on some lighthearted leisure trip. It could have been an outing with close friends back home—a trip to the hot springs for a swim or a hike in the hills of Mount Tamalpais. And I was included in their jokes, feeling that I'd been really accepted into the team.

At one point in the afternoon, when I was starting to feel tired and less sure-footed than normal, I slipped on some slippery gravel, landed on my derrière, and bounced back up, half-hoping no one would notice.

"Mary Anne Didi, *arum gaarnu man laagyo?*" quipped Bhim Raj, our jokester cook. *Do you want to rest?* Gentle chuckles from everyone.

"Ah, Bhim Raj wants to carry you!" retorted Sita, to more snickering.

"Okay, *bholi*, Bhim Raj? *Tik?*" I responded over his protestations. *Tomorrow, OK?* Raucous laughter.

Nepalis are more ready to laugh, to poke fun, to enjoy the simplest aspects of everyday life than any people I've ever encountered. That lightheartedness had helped me to cope with the challenges of this job—at least on those days when I was successful at coping—as nothing else did.

Just as it was getting dark, we stopped on a small treeless hill close to a river and set up camp. The nearby hamlet, Kamantar, consisted of a dozen or so stone houses scattered along the trail. After the porters set up the tents, we relaxed over dinner sitting in a circle near the top of the hill, under a bright half-moon.

And what a change from our usual arrival scene: Because we were spending that night outside the main village center, there had been no advance notice of our coming. No crowds gathering to greet us, no curious children poking their heads into my tent, no villagers lined up with requests for medicine. Just one evening of peace, and it was a blessed relief.

Excusing myself immediately after dinner, I crawled into my gray-green cocoon for the night. Resting against my backpack, I opened my journal. The light from the kerosene lamp that flickered on the open pages in front of me was calming, almost mesmerizing. I was too tired to either read or write, but also not ready for sleep. Well-worn advice from Baba Ram Das, guru to many in my generation, echoed in my ears: *Be here now. Be where you are now, not anywhere else.*

Crickets were calling out a steady, strangely lulling babble. From the tea shop nearby, men were chatting about the day's events. The sounds of children playing were like those of children anywhere, and only vaguely did it register that they were shouting in Nepali, playing Nepali games. Someone beyond the tea shop was tuning in snatches of folk music on a transistor radio. Farther down the hill I heard the rhythmic thumping of a family's grain mill, doubtless a woman trying to get a head start on the next day's work. In their nearby tent, Sita and Sushila quibbled over the vaccine arrangements for the next day. I slumped down farther onto my sleeping bag. Every cell in my body was alive, buzzing pleasantly. The world around me was exactly as it should be—warm, harmonious. Maybe this was a life I could live.

Part way through our first day in Borlang, I looked up to see the headman of the area approaching. He was tall and serious-looking, wearing western clothes, as most of the village leaders did. Something about his determined strides told me that he was coming with a request, perhaps a big one.

"Memsaab, my neighbor's wife is very sick," he began. "Maybe you have medicine that would help her?" He was polite but spoke with the air of a man who was used to being heard. At his side was the neighbor, a disheveled-looking man in his late forties who shifted restlessly, a look of shock mixed with fear in his eyes.

I asked about the woman's symptoms, and when it seemed likely that it was a serious issue, the three of us set off for the man's house. I learned on the way that his wife, Maya, was around twenty-eight years old and they had no children. *Was she pregnant?* He hesitated. *Yes, maybe,* he said. She had gotten a tetanus shot from our team during a previous visit to Borlang some two months prior. Not long after, she thought she was pregnant, attributing it to the "medicine" we gave her. Then, early that morning, she had sudden abdominal pain, so severe she could barely speak or move, and was getting weaker all the time.

I followed the chief and his friend a short distance to a small thatched-roof house where a very pale young woman lay in the shade on the open porch. Several village women huddled around her, holding her hands, with worried looks. They moved aside as I knelt beside her on the straw mat. Maya's lips and ears had a milky pale sheen and she was damp with perspiration, moaning and whispering words I couldn't understand.

"Didi," I said gently, taking her hand. "*Kasto chha? Kahaa dukhyo?*" *How are you? Where does it hurt?* She pointed weakly at her abdomen, and her arm dropped back to her side. I slid my hand gently under her wrinkled cotton cummerbund and felt a rigid, board-like abdomen underneath. A bad sign. Her pulse was a very rapid, thready tapping that told me she was going into shock.

"*Dheri dukhyo,*" an older women beside me said, looking at me with sad, questioning eyes. *She hurts a lot.* I nodded and felt a surge of sympathy not only for Maya, but also for the whole group of concerned friends and relatives who were sharing her suffering. The sour scent of anxiety, of helpless fear, filled the air around us.

But I was there because I was expected to help. My clinical training propelled me through the most likely causes of her condition. Although there were several possibilities, at the top of the list was a ruptured ectopic pregnancy, when the embryo settles in the fallopian tubes instead of the uterus. As it grows, it bursts the thin tube walls. This diagnosis was even more likely when I thought about how old she was to be childless. Infertility is sometimes caused by scarred tubes, which may have led to her condition. Even if that wasn't the cause, something bad had happened internally and, if she could be saved, it would require surgery very quickly.

"Ke garne?" That question, posed by the village chief, was on everyone's mind. I looked around at the gathered villagers. All eyes were on me.

I knew of only two realistic choices. They could transport Maya to the district's Protestant mission hospital, around an eight-hour walk away. It was a well-run hospital with basic surgical capacity, something the government hospital, which was a mere four hours away, didn't have. If she arrived in time and if the surgeon was there, an operation could save her life.

Those ifs, I thought. The chance of success was very slight, but I was sure she wouldn't survive the day without treatment. I didn't even have pain medication strong enough to ease her suffering. The other choice: Bring on the traditional healer, gather the family, say prayers, make offerings, and when she died, mourn yet another maternal death.

The implications of either option weighed heavily.

What should I say? If something was to be done, it needed to be done very quickly. Could they get her over the steep trails to the hospital? Would this trip make her suffering even worse? I worried about giving hope where there was none, causing more pain, when acceptance of a sad reality might be the kinder course.

But I'd worked for several years in emergency rooms in the US dealing with this kind of urgent, life-threatening condition. One evening a woman was brought in with similar symptoms. Within minutes of the diagnosis of an ectopic pregnancy, she was prepped for surgery and sent off for what turned out to be a fairly routine operation. A pint or two of blood, a couple of days in the hospital, and she was home again, sad at losing her pregnancy, but physically intact. That was the option that I wanted for Maya. Maybe it was possible.

Her husband looked at me expectantly, and we stepped away from the main group of onlookers to speak in low tones.

"Sir, your wife is very sick," I said to him, swallowing between sentences. "She may die if she doesn't have an operation."

Sita had arrived by then, slightly breathless, her forehead damp with perspiration after a rapid trip from the camp. She stood beside me, providing an occasional explanation to the men if they seemed uncertain about something I'd said. However, my message was not complicated: I thought Maya was bleeding inside, and the only treatment possible would be for her to have surgery to stop the bleeding. If they could get her to the local mission hospital, maybe she could be saved. *Maybe*, I repeated several times.

Maya's husband looked at me, seemingly bewildered at this information. A lengthy discussion with the chief and neighborhood men ensued. She was so sick, could the doctor really help her? Wasn't there something else that could be done? But after much debate, they agreed to transport her to the hospital.

The first plan was to load her sitting upright into a *doko*, the cone-shaped basket used for hauling goods that was also used to transport sick people. Then it would be the husband's job to carry her. I quickly explained that she needed to lie flat, so her blood could circulate to her head; that would require making a stretcher. More discussion. How many men would it take to carry her on a stretcher? Who could spare the day or two it would take for them to be away from their work? How would they make the device?

As the men negotiated, I knelt by the young woman, even paler now, to check her pulse and try to reassure her.

"We're taking you to the hospital, Didi," I said, leaning close to be sure she could hear me. I hoped that if she were alert enough to understand, she would find comfort in that plan. However, I also knew that "hospital" was a last resort for most village Nepalis, undertaken rarely and only when other options had been exhausted. She didn't respond and perhaps didn't even register what I was saying.

For the next hour, I circled the throng, trying to understand what was being done and why it was taking so long. *Why is nothing happening? Don't they get it?* I agonized. An hour or two of delay could mean the difference between saving her life and losing it.

Although there was nothing I could do but wait, the burden of her care seemed to rest on my shoulders, and it was heavy. Every nerve in my body seemed activated, every muscle on alert. I was the nurse in charge, responsible for seeing that things were done quickly, efficiently. But I'd never been faced with this kind of challenge. I needed backup, but there was no protocol, no on-call doctors, no surgical team, no emergency cart. And no chaplain to call when everything else failed.

Finally, the crowd moved aside as Maya's husband and another man approached the house with a cleverly contrived stretcher of rope and wooden poles.

"Ah, that's good," I commented to no one in particular. They laid the stretcher on a flat spot on the ground by the porch and placed a heavy blanket on top. I helped the men lift the sick woman, straw mat and all, onto the device. She moaned as she was settled onto the stretcher. Her husband leaned over and spoke to her softly, and she gave an even softer moan in response. When he stood back up, his face was grave but had a new look of determination. An older woman from the gathering stepped back up to whisper something to her, and everyone moved off the porch to give the men room.

Three volunteers would help the woman's husband carry the stretcher. They took their positions, one at each corner and, after a few false starts, hoisted it up and moved into the sunlight. She cried out briefly as the men shifted her position to even the load, startling the crowd. The older woman, Maya's mother, stepped up to give her daughter's hand a farewell touch. Her deeply lined face was a study in sadness.

At last the four men began the long trek down the path and out of sight. Gradually the gathered villagers drifted away, with somber looks and muttered conversations. I began taking deep, slow breaths, trying to release the tension that had been growing all that afternoon. I suddenly felt an overwhelming exhaustion.

By that time, most of my team had arrived to see what was happening, and we returned together to camp. The two vaccinators asked me what had made the woman so sick. I explained the basic information about an ectopic pregnancy.

"No one really knows why this problem happens," I said. Their puzzled looks didn't disappear.

Then Sita said to me softly, "The neighbors are worried that someone put an evil spell on her, Mary Anne Didi."

I gave myself a mental smack on the forehead. Of course. No matter how often I had heard Nepali stories of how supernatural forces caused illness, I would forget that perspective and revert to my biomedical thinking when I was with a sick individual. They had been skeptical about what "modern" medicine could do for this problem, and thus the lengthy discussions about how to respond. Why go to the hospital when Western doctors don't know how to treat supernatural problems? They were understandably doubtful about the hospital services, too, because good care was so rarely available in rural areas.

Yet, somehow, my advice to transport the woman for care had prevailed. My burden felt even heavier, and I held on ever more tightly to hope that she would survive. *Will they make it on time?* I asked myself for the rest of that afternoon, over and over. Was it the right decision to advise them to go? What if she dies—would the tetanus shot be blamed, as immunizations sometimes were when unusual problems followed the injection? Looking back, I can see that there had been no "right" decision, that either choice would have had a similar outcome. But at the time, I felt compelled to try everything possible to fix the problem, to help this unfortunate young woman beat the odds.

We finished work and had an uneasy supper, gathered on mats in a dark room near the cooking fire. The flickering flames reflected somber, thoughtful faces. Joking and chatter were sparse now, and I imagined that the others had the same thoughts. *What happened to her? When will we know?*

After the meal, as we were about to move into the adjoining room to prepare for tomorrow's work, I heard a man's voice conversing with a porter just outside. Sita went out to join them and returned moments later with a solemn expression, a little frown, and half-closed eyes. She glanced around the room, waiting for silence.

"She died in Taple—about halfway to the hospital. They've come back," was all Sita said.

Murmurs of dismay and sympathy rippled through the room. I felt a sudden thud in my chest, my fears confirmed. *What can I say?*

"Oh, how sad. It was just too late to help her," I told the team, feeling the need to comfort them as well as myself. There was scant comfort for any of us in those words, though. I turned and made my way slowly back to my tent.

I slumped onto my sleeping bag. The poor woman, who died in such misery. I could do so little to help her or her distressed husband. Was it bad judgment to send them off on a journey to the hospital that was probably fruitless? Should I have accepted their hesitation to fight back against a death that was probably inevitable?

Many years later I still wondered what I would have done, given the choice again, on that afternoon in Borlang. Helping people was what I did, starting early in life as I took charge of my younger siblings when we were growing up, and continuing with my career as a nurse. Deciding what really helped and what didn't was not a decision I'd ever had to make. This was a new lesson, and one I hoped wouldn't be repeated.

Another unsettling thought nagged at me: As close as I felt to my friends on the team, the limited possibilities for treatment that Maya faced would have been the same if it had been Sita who had gotten so ill. The options for most Nepali women were very few. Yet, if it was I who had fallen off a cliff or had a sudden attack of appendicitis, there would have been an immediate effort to get word to our office in Kathmandu, and a medical helicopter would be dispatched to fly me to care. The chasm between them and me was enormous. Maya's crisis showed me the stark face of the extent of that privilege, and it was deeply unsettling.

Daily life in Gorkha brought me face-to-face with inequities that I'd never had to acknowledge so directly before. The vast gaps in power between men and women, upper castes and lower castes, those with more land and those with less were ever-present. In Kathmandu, the contrast was even starker: The royal family and members of the former ruling class, the Ranas, lived in enormous mansions and traveled the world in limousines and personal jets. Yet the men and women who brought them wood for their fires and food for their feasts were ragged and barefoot, with malnourished children at home. After working in low-income areas in the US, I'd thought I understood poverty. But here I couldn't avoid seeing these even deeper inequalities, an extreme I had never before experienced.

I learned another humbling lesson that day in Borlang. Even with practically no drugs or equipment, I could recognize serious medical conditions and recommend interventions. But most of the problems of a Nepali villager went far beyond figuring out a medical response. Part of my job was to recognize the limits to what I could do and connect with the collective wisdom of a people who had been dealing with these challenges for centuries. Sometimes I could help, but other times the Nepali traditions and systems for coping were more realistic —and more humane—than anything I had to offer.

Chapter 15

Storybook Tales

Finally, the monsoon rains were really over, and the snowy tips of the Himals regularly peeked out at points along the trail. The hillsides were a brilliant green, with terraced rice fields that could have been lush, deep backyard lawns someone had neglected to mow.

After a short break at the Gorkha house, I was with my team headed for Tandrung. I was in the groove, not talking much but enjoying the slightly cooler weather and clear blue skies. I was fascinated by the dozens of butterflies that darted along the trail with us, soaking in the sun just as we were. Sometimes I lagged behind the others, savoring every peaceful moment of the bucolic scenes we wandered through.

The villages we passed by seemed more quaint and picturesque than ever. *I could be in a folktale right now,* I thought, walking down a shady lane through a tiny village with thatched roofs over reddish-brown cottages, cows grazing here and there. The fences between fields were cleverly woven of prickly shrubs, the branches woven tightly together. They were sometimes connected by stiles, those ladder-like devices for climbing over fences I'd only seen in children's books. There was no sign of wheeled vehicles anywhere, not even a donkey cart. And an astounding lack of anything resembling trash. *These folks must be the original recyclers!* I marveled. No piles of paper, bottles, cans, old clothes, or worn-out toys. Everything was used and used again, or not necessary in the first place.

We passed women carrying water home on their heads in elegant brass containers. Kids chattered happily on their way to school, little girls wearing dark-blue skirts, boys in the same color of pants, and most of them with surprisingly white shirts. *How do they ever stay that clean?* I wondered, knowing that village women had to carry their precious water from sources that might be an hour or more away from the house. My daily sponge bath in the tent always seemed a futile effort to delay the inevitable chalky red dust that settled on every surface by midmorning.

Several women stopped to stare as we passed by.

"*Eh, kahile aaunuu bhayo?*" they chirped cheerfully, smiling at our entourage but most interested in me, the foreigner. *When did you come?* As with all simple pleasantries, almost any answer would do.

"*Ahile, didi, ahile!*" I replied, laughing back. *Just now!* A few more questions followed about where we were headed and why. I noticed two younger girls, teenagers, with their heads together in whispered giggles as they looked at me. I knew they were asking that familiar question—is that a woman or a man? I still wore a skirt just below the knee and a T-shirt, typical of what Nepali men wore. By now I'd been through this many times.

"*Aaimaai!*" I said, sticking out my chest and pulling back my hair so they could see my gold-tooled Nepali earrings. *Woman!*

The girls shrieked with appreciation, and we passed on down the path. A group of schoolboys greeted us next with shouts in carefully enunciated staccato English: "Where-are-you-go-ing? Where-did-you-come-from?"

The boys seemed pleased with an answer that they recognized: "Tandrung!" and even more delighted at hearing that we had come from Gorkha village.

"Gorkha *baata? Bhaisi manche!*" they shouted with glee. Water buffalo, *bhaisi*, are the slowest beasts around, and they couldn't believe that it was already nearly noon and we'd only gotten as far as their village. But all of us, the heavily laden porters, the sari'd vaccinators and slowpoke me, were all enjoying the leisurely day.

Two of the porters leaned forward and walked with a swaying motion, mimicking the *bhaisi*, as we headed out of the village. The boys shrieked again in appreciation.

Finally arriving at the Tandrung village center, we sank gratefully onto the base of the stone *chautara* under a massive peepal tree and waited for the village leader to arrive to give us formal permission to work in his village. Within minutes we were surrounded by a crowd of villagers, mostly women and kids, fascinated to watch us as we just . . . sat there. The headman arrived eventually, wearing western clothes and relatively young for a village leader. He made a few welcoming remarks and then was on his way.

Though a bit more enthusiasm would have been welcome, in fact the assistance of the *kadwal*, the town crier, was probably more essential. I was always fascinated by the very existence of this medieval figure, who had a booming voice and whose job was to announce village events by going to a few critical spots and shouting a brief message at the top of his lungs. In this case it would be a bellowing, sing-song, "Bring all small children to the *chautara* tomorrow morning for their injec-shun." Within an hour we could hear a distant voice shouting the message from the highest hill near the village: "*Subbai saano buccha-haaru bholi bihanna ler-AU-nu-os. . . .*"

The *kadwal's* efforts seemed to be successful, and we had a good turnout for immunizations the next day. With the help of Ram Lal, our "writing porter," Sita and I finished with the last screaming child by midafternoon and gathered up our supplies for the return to camp. We had barely begun the three-hour hike back when someone called to us from lower on the trail. It was a man carrying a young boy about five or six years old, his wife trailing behind. We stopped and waited for them to catch up.

"Memsaab, my son has a very painful leg," the man said to me, sounding anxious and shy at the same time. "I heard you were here for the injections. Can you help him?"

He put the boy down onto the ground and pointed at the problem area: a huge abscess swelling up the front of the boy's thigh, clearly a painful pocket of infection. The boy looked at me with wide, frightened eyes, too miserable to even cry. His nose was running with the perennial cold that Nepali children always seemed to have. His clothes were nearly solid with dirt, but I had long since given up feeling critical of unwashed children or clothing: I'd found out how difficult it was for me to stay clean even for a day, even when water was carried directly to my tent. Still, the dust and dirt made skin infections a common problem, especially for young children.

Though the conditions on the trail weren't ideal, the abscess needed to be drained, and there was no need to bring the child back to camp. I had what I needed—a knife, gauze, alcohol to cleanse the site, and a few days' worth of antibiotic tablets to send with them. Releasing the infected material was the main solution to this very common problem, even when sometimes carried out with my trusty Swiss Army knife.

A short distance up the trail we arranged ourselves on a rock bench that served as a travelers' rest. Both parents held the little boy tightly as I cleaned the knife blade and prepared to lance the abscess. The only sound was my voice, telling him quietly what a good boy he was, how much better he would feel when I was done. He whimpered slightly and to my relief, barely moved as I proceeded.

"Tik! Siddhiyo!" Okay! Done, I said, smiling brightly as I finished. The boy gave a faint grimace of relief as Sita stepped up to pop a hard candy into his mouth. Everyone seemed to relax instantly. I instructed the parents in giving the antibiotic and applying warm compresses for the next few days to be sure the wound continued to drain.

As we finished, I thought back to the recent tragedy with poor Maya and felt another twinge of regret and sadness that I wasn't able to help her. *At least I get to do something useful today,* I thought. A sense of accomplishment came from a simple procedure like this, even if it would relieve only this one little person's suffering.

We were preparing to set off again for camp when the boy's father began a conversation with Sita. She turned to me. "Mary Anne Didi, do you want to hear him play?" she asked. "This man is a *gaini*, and he wants to thank you for your help by playing for you."

A *gaini*! I knew of them but had never met nor heard one, this Nepali version of a wandering minstrel. A fabulous end to the day.

"Of course! That would be great!" I enthused, with a wide grin.

The *gaini* pulled from his rough canvas pack a small violin-like instrument that had been carved out of one piece of wood. The central portion was hollow, with three strings that were tethered onto the neck by wooden pegs. He used a simple bow that looked like it might have been made of the tail hairs of a horse. "*Mero saraangi,*" he said, simply naming his instrument, and began.

For the next ten or fifteen minutes the man sang and played an enchanting rhythmic music that made me at first think of Appalachian hill songs. It had a sing-song quality, telling stories and making observations about his world. Though I assumed the songs were traditional folk music, I realized after a time that many of the lyrics were improvised, referring to local events that even included the arrival of an immunization team in Tandrung. The "Memsaab" was in the music too. Sita and Ram Lal looked at each other and at me, grinning.

I listened with fascination as the *gaini's* music filled the air. Foreign as the tunes were, they were also somehow familiar. I grew up loving country fiddler's tunes and recognized some of the same sounds in the twang of the *saraangi*. In my talented family, music was an important part of every gathering. Suddenly, home seemed not so far away.

We sat quietly, enjoying the serenade while cool breezes chased away the heat of the afternoon sun. *What a gift,* I thought. I was overwhelmed with a feeling of connectedness with this little corner of the world. I'd come to Nepal to experience a new place, a different culture, but the more time I spent in these hills, the more I realized I had in common with the people who lived here.

The *gaini* stopped, and we asked for one more song. By the time he finished, the sun was getting lower in the afternoon sky, so we gave our thanks and, because this was his primary livelihood, offered the man a few rupee notes.

The trail back to camp was an exhausting slog. But the heat of the day had abated, and we made it back in less than the expected two hours. As we approached my tent, the sun nearly out of sight, I wanted nothing more than to pull off my tennis shoes and sink onto my sleeping bag. But before I reached the tent flap, Dil Man came up to me with a worried look.

"Mary Anne Didi, Prem is very sick. Can you get him some medicine?" he asked.

"*Taauko duukyo?*" I asked. *A headache?* Prem, the cook for this trek, was prone to migraine headaches. That would be quick, some aspirin and hope that he could sleep it off.

"Yes," he answered, and then hesitated. "But the *jhaakri* has come too." *Oh, this should be interesting,* I mused. Jhaakris are one of the traditional healers who connect with the spirit world to treat illness. I hadn't yet seen this kind of Nepali healer, despite many queries about what they did and how. I wasn't so tired that I would miss the opportunity to see one in action.

We moved into a room in the village meeting house where Prem had set up the kitchen. He was lying on a mat in the mostly dark room, half-sitting against a duffel bag and holding his head in obvious pain. The other porters were gathered around him, wearing sympathetic frowns. At one side stood an older man I didn't know who looked intently at Prem, saying something unintelligible. He held something in one hand that looked like a long feather duster. *The jhaakri?* I thought. *Not very exotic-looking.* Pictures I had seen of *jhaakris* in action had them dressed in traditional outfits with headdresses and heavy necklaces; this person was indistinguishable from the other village men.

He glanced up at me briefly and then continued his repetitive murmuring in a low voice. After a short time, he began "sweeping" Prem with the broom, beginning at his head and moving toward his feet, blowing puffs of air on him at intervals and chanting the same incantation over and over.

When the *jhaakri* had completed his efforts, he muttered something to the porters and unceremoniously left the room. No loud pronouncements, no closing ceremony. I was reminded of physicians I had worked with whose confident manner with patients was so low-key and understated that they were occasionally mistaken for orderlies.

"Better now, Prem?" asked one of the porters.

"Yes, I think so," he replied weakly. Then, seeing me in the doorway, he said with a little moan, "Memsaab, could you bring me medicine too? It's very bad today."

Sita came up behind me and whispered, "The *jhaakri* said he swept out the spirit that's causing the headache. Maybe Prem will be okay now. But I think some aspirin will help too."

I gave the Nepali affirmative ears-to-shoulders nod and stepped back outside. It seemed a reasonable request. The *jhaakri*'s ministrations might help, but why not use everything at hand?

I was impressed with the ability of many of the Nepalis I met to reconcile two very different ways of seeing the world. For example,

Sita's work with us, providing immunizations to prevent childhood illnesses, contrasted with a much more complicated set of beliefs in how health and illness worked. In Nepal, poor health could be caused by a wide range of spiritual and other causes. But it seemed logical, particularly in this setting of relative scarcity, to use more than one type of treatment when illness struck. "Medical pluralism," a term used by anthropologists, in practice often meant embracing what was available and hoping it worked. I had discussed this topic with Dr. K. C., and even he admitted he was never sure of how much the spirit world affected the results of his efforts.

I retrieved three aspirin from our medicine box and gave them to Dil Man to deliver. A cute, gangly young guy, he was still in late adolescence and eager to please. I smiled as he grinned and rushed off with his important task.

One of the other porters would cook for Prem tonight, so I was able to slip into the tent and onto my sleeping bag for the luxury of a nap until dinnertime. I found myself fighting sleep, wanting to think about the day's events. A *kadwal*, a *gaini,* and a *jhaakri* all in one day, I mused, with a flush of satisfaction. And then, confusion: Just when I think I can't bear this life anymore, a captivating day like today comes along.

Chapter 16

Dashain!

The biggest festival of them all was about to begin all over the country: Dashain, the harvest festival. Since it was pointless to try to work during major holidays, especially this one, we were headed for a ten-day break in Kathmandu.

For a much-anticipated event, Sita would accompany Corinne for her first visit to the city and spend part of the holiday there. We were both dying to be with Sita when she had her first taste of urban life, a world she'd heard about, but in all her twenty-some years had never experienced.

Sita and Corinne would leave from the Gorkha house, and Krishna and I with a local porter would go directly from our camp in Tandrung, through a neighboring district. I was told it would be a nine- or ten-hour day.

Leaving camp, my trekking day started off badly. A couple of days earlier, wearing my usual flip-flops, I'd raked my small toe against a rock, and now it was red, swollen, and very tender. Although I usually wore tennis shoes on longer treks, that was not going to work for this one. I wasn't particularly worried, though, as I had worn my flip-flops for most trekking days. What I hadn't factored in was that these were new sandals, not yet broken in, with a slightly rough, patterned surface where my sole met the sandal to make them less slippery.

Krishna and I charged off into the clear, cool morning. We chatted for a while, then strode on quietly with birdsong and the squeaking of our packs the only sounds. Gradually the soles of my feet began to burn, slightly, then with a stinging urgency. By the time we had been on the trail three hours, each step felt like I was walking on burning coals. The patterned surface of the sandal acted like sandpaper, and by the end of the day I would have massive blisters on the soles of both feet.

I cursed silently with every step, trying to dream up an alternative to this torture. I called out to Krishna.

"Krishna, my feet are really sore. These new sandals. Any ideas what I can do?" I asked.

"On, Mary Anne Didi, so sorry! We have a long way to go today. Do you want to put on your tennis shoes?" he replied, calling to the porter who carried my bag to stop.

We unpacked the *doko*, retrieved the shoes, and I gingerly slipped them on. Within five steps I groaned even more loudly. Now the entire injured foot hurt, not just the soles. Back to the flip-flops.

The rest of the day involved another ten hours of walking. Ten . . . more . . . hours, each step more painful than the last. At one point where the path was flat and dusty, I tried walking barefoot. No better. Then I tried prancing along mostly on my heels, to spare the more painful soles, but that only worked for a short time. The searing, burning sensation on my soles seemed to travel up both legs, and I started to worry about a worsening infection from the small injury responsible for this agony.

With every step I cursed my stupidity for having only my new flip-flops along, for not keeping my trusty, broken-in ones handy, for wearing flip-flops in the first place instead of tennis shoes. But there was nothing to do except keep going.

At long last, we arrived just after dark in the tiny village of Palpa. It had only two establishments, one a very small shop and the other a low-budget teahouse-restaurant-lodge where we would eat and spend the night.

"Finally!" I groaned to Krishna. I limped behind him as he moved toward the teahouse to make the arrangements.

The ancient-appearing proprietor was barely four feet tall, but she smiled freely and gave sympathetic murmurings at hearing about my sore feet. She quickly served a standard *dal bhat* dinner to the three of us, which we ate in the crowded tea stall, and then ushered me up a narrow staircase to a tiny room with two benches covered by straw mats. That was it for the "lodge" accommodations: no beds, no quilts, no mosquito netting, and certainly no toilet facilities. But hey, the cost included the meal, and all I really wanted was to get off and stay off my feet, so I didn't complain. Krishna brought up a sleeping bag, which I rolled out, lying on top and hoping it would be a barrier against the fleas that likely infested those straw mats. Tossing and turning on the hard bench, I somehow slept.

The highway was still two hours away, I learned the next morning. But by then I was oblivious to all but the anticipation of transport back to Kathmandu. In one of those miraculously well-timed rescues, by the time we crossed the final bridge, the Foundation jeep was there, waiting to pick us up. I thought I'd never again feel such relief as that moment of sinking onto the back seat, feet throbbing but spared from further battering.

I spent the first few days back in Kathmandu in my room, tending to my sore feet and luxuriating on my deep foam mattress in the quiet comfort of the Chabahil house. I read, wrote letters, and soaked my blisters, waiting for them to heal enough that I could walk again without pain.

Sita had arrived with Corinne the day before me, and I was anxious to see and hear her impressions of this messy, busy city. It was Sita's first time for virtually everything: first ride in a car, first electricity and indoor plumbing, first paved streets, and first really modern house.

They burst into my room the morning after I arrived. Sita sat down on the bed beside me, breathless and bright-eyed in a flowered blue sari, her hair in her usual neatly braided bun. "Oh, Mary Anne Didi, Corinne told me about your feet!" were her first words. She had to inspect my wounds, cluck in sympathy, and offer suggestions for how to heal them faster. Sita was always a comforting presence. But I was impatient to hear about her first big-city experience.

"Sita, tell me about your trip!" I demanded, as soon as the discussion of the blisters had wrapped up. "What do you think about this place? Is it what you expected? What do you like best?"

Corinne beamed with pride at being Sita's designated tour guide. "Oh, she LOVES it!" she said. "Don't you, Sita?" she added. They'd just had a tour of Bodnath, the important Buddhist temple nearby, and Corinne had shown her around our luxurious residence.

Sita looked at us, first one and then the other, shaking her head slowly with an expression that was a blend of surprise and disbelief.

"It's not how I thought it would be," she said, finally. "It's very noisy, isn't it?" Her eyes had a bemused, searching look, as if at a loss to describe and categorize all she was seeing for the first time. "But I like it, yes," she concluded. "This house is so big. It's beautiful. Several families could live here." Sita looked around at the elegant mahogany closet and bounced appreciatively on the soft foam mattress.

Then she gave us a searching look and asked a question I had anticipated with dread: "Is your home in America this like?"

That inquiry, innocent as it was, fell like a blow. Here was our Sita, for the first time coming face-to-face with the stark inequalities in her own country and trying to understand how far they went. *Does the whole rest of the world live like this?* I could imagine her thinking.

It was a subject that I'd tried to avoid discussing since my first days in Gorkha: the almost unimaginable gulf between what we had in America and the material world of rural Nepal. Sometimes it came out as a very personal concern. Although educated Nepalis usually understood that asking questions related to wealth or income was not acceptable in Western cultures, the rural population wasn't familiar with such niceties. During one of my first weeks in Gorkha, I'd had that very conversation when chatting with the vaccinators.

"We work very hard for our pay, and it's only 2800 rupees a month," Sita had commented then, which was roughly $180. "We would really like an increase. How much do you nurses make?"

Gulp. Though we were "volunteers," we'd just had a raise in stipend to $250 a month, plus food and lodging fully covered. Even if that monthly allowance would seem meager back home, here the difference of $70 a month for them could mean having a few luxuries rather than only the essentials—a new bangle now and then, or meat for a special meal.

I'd stuttered a bit in response, then replied that our salary was a little more, but about the same. That simple question blared a big truth at me: how different my life would always be from theirs, solely by virtue of where I was born. Now, as I tried to see Kathmandu through Sita's eyes, that discomfort returned.

Fortunately, Corinne jumped in with a gentle deflection of the question. "Oh, this is fancier than how most of us live in America," she said. "A few do, but not most of us." Sita nodded, though I could see by her thoughtful frown that the question wasn't really resolved. Changing the subject, Corinne asked what Sita wanted to do with the rest of her day.

Just then Maya, the charming maid whom I'd met on my very first day in that house, stepped into the room and asked if Sita wanted to come down to the kitchen to chat. Sita jumped up and followed her out the door, anxious, I imagined, to get a sense of how a Nepali woman like her could live in such a strange yet exciting place.

Corinne quickly filled me in about Sita's experience thus far: her dazed response to the first ride in the office car, her startled reactions at the honking of horns and the sight of massive trucks on the highway. Once in Kathmandu, she'd begun asking questions of every Nepali she met about the practicalities of living in the city, about jobs, the cost of apartments, and how they coped with getting around. The bus system fascinated her.

"We're going this afternoon to the bazaar for her to buy a footlocker. It's for carrying her things when she moves to Kathmandu, I'm sure," was Corinne's assessment.

I gasped. "Really? Do you think that's what she's thinking?" I was taken aback and began to wonder if we'd done Sita a favor by helping her have this experience. "Would she ever want to move here?"

"Maybe. Sita's always looking around at other ways to live, isn't she?" Corinne replied.

It was true. The simple fact that she was in her late twenties and unmarried meant that Sita would not settle for what her entire society expected of her, despite more social pressures to do so than I could even imagine. Sita was her own person, and she was respected for it. At the same time, I couldn't see her being happy living in Kathmandu, away from the community that was so intrinsic to her life in Gorkha.

As we sent Sita off on a bus back to Gorhka, I could only hope that what we'd shown her would help her feel confident in the path she'd chosen. Or would she always long for more, now that she'd seen this new world?

We were in Kathmandu for two weeks of the big Dashain holiday, with a different celebration every day. The traditions range from kite flying and card playing to ornately decorated homes, new clothes for everyone, and legendary feasting after the sacrifice of chickens, goats, or buffalo—notable in a country where meat eating was not routine among most of the impoverished population.

I had my usual curiosity about what this event meant to my Nepali friends, who lived every year in anticipation of the fall Dashain holiday. In the fields in Gorkha I'd seen evidence of why kids loved the holiday: the skeletons of *pings*, large wooden constructions that, with planks added as seats when the celebrations were under way, became Ferris wheels.

"It's like your Christmas," I was told. But the only specifics I could get out of Sita about any deeper meaning was that it was a celebration of good over evil. Most of what she described related to the customs and activities, the fun, the gifts, the feasting. *Yep, like Christmas*, I thought. Later I found that, according to Hindu religious writings, the festival marks victory over an evil demon and a demon-king who cruelly terrorized India in the form of a raging water buffalo. The goddess Durga was helpful in winning these victories, so she is particularly worshiped during Dashain.

One of the big Dashain days took place after I was back on my feet: the ritual sacrifice of thousands of animals at holy places, with accompanying prayers and other rituals, the *pujah*. I was squeamish at the thought of what I'd see. Though I ate meat, it was from a grocery store—widely, safely separated from that living animal it had once been. Even the beef cattle we raised on the family ranch were never slaughtered for our meals, but sold to be fattened and butchered elsewhere, mostly appearing on our table as hamburger. But this was too important an event to miss.

On the crisp, bright morning of the big public event, I set out on my bike for the central stadium for the public sacrifice of goats, buffalo, and sheep. After pedaling only a few blocks, it became clear that this was a Kathmandu I'd never seen before. Masses of people swarmed the streets in their brightly colored finery—moms, dads, and kids on their way to a temple or to visit family. That was what I expected. What I didn't anticipate was what I saw and heard and felt in the air: the terror of the goats of Kathmandu. Thousands had been brought in from the countryside and sold to householders for their *pujahs*. Every street was filled with their wild and plaintive bleating as they were led off, fighting against their lead ropes, to become part of the celebration. The vaguely metallic smell of blood combined with the stench of some goats' panic-induced diarrhea and the sight of a few bloody remains of the early sacrifices gave me a sickening feeling. I wanted to turn around and go home, leave all this, go to my safe, sheltering room and forget what was happening around me.

But there was meaning here for millions of Nepalis. I was determined to get a sense of it, so I charged ahead on my bike to a huge arena-sized courtyard. The crowds coming and going were massive, but I elbowed my way to an upper level of the seating until I could see the activities on the ground below. Armed troops stood at attention along an entire wall, and opposite them a military band tooted out the occasional stirring anthem. Dozens of young water buffaloes were lined up at one end of the arena. A few men milled busily about the field, at the center of which was a line of Nepali flags and brass plates of food and flowers that were part of the ceremony. There was a general sense of confusion and disorder, but anticipation as well.

In the center of the grounds, with the others at a respectful distance, stood the executioner, holding a *kukri*, a giant sword-knife, in his hands. He eyed the young buffalo calf that was tied to a peg in the ground directly in front of him and waved the *kukri* up and down, like a batter preparing to swing. Suddenly, with one decisive hack of the knife that was too quick to actually see, the animal's head dropped freely to the ground, its body following suit in the opposite direction. I heard a faint "Ooh" from the crowd. Then two men jumped forward and dragged the headless carcass by the back legs, encircling the flags and *pujah* materials with a faint trail of blood.

It happened so fast I could barely register my reaction. When I realized what I'd just seen, a question sprang into my mind: What on earth does this signify? I remembered that Dashain was celebrating victory over a demon in the form of a raging water buffalo. *Is that what this is about?* I wondered. They kill the demon, and then can enjoy the feast that results. It was as good an explanation as any.

Whatever the meaning, the sacrificial act was an impressive feat, impossible-looking enough that it could have been a magic trick. It was to go on for several hours that day, with goats and sheep all having their turns. For me, however, once was enough. I'd done it, I'd seen the event, and I wanted nothing more than to go home and put all this gore and mayhem out of my mind.

As I stowed my bicycle back at the house, I could see that something significant was about to take place.

"What's going on?" I asked Corinne, who had her camera out on the dining room table and was cleaning its lenses.

"Remember, the office *pujah* is today too!" she replied, clearly excited at the idea. Corinne was always seeking out cultural aspects of the Nepali world, and here it was, coming to us. Our own *pujah.* "Gopal and the others are going to cut a goat and bless all the Foundation vehicles."

Right, kill a goat to bless the vehicles. Okay, why not? Catholics had the Pope bless the fleet every year. And yet, my mind rebelled, the images from the stadium rolling around in my head. A bloody blessing really didn't make sense, didn't fit into the world I knew. I brought back the mantra I'd used over and over again in dealing with the strange and unfamiliar: *This is Nepal. Accept it.*

We all stepped out into the bright but chilly backyard of the compound. The office cars, hoods raised in anticipation of this annual blessing, were arranged in a row in the back alley. Bowls filled with flowers, fruit, rice, and brilliant crimson and gold tika powder were arranged on a stone wall nearby. A young goat, tethered by a small rope and looking calm and unconcerned, nosed around at the green grass.

The Brahmin priest who had been summoned to conduct the *pujah* gathered the male Nepali staff and began a lengthy ceremony. All of us, including the goat, were blessed with a *tika* on our foreheads and a *malla*, a necklace of flowers. The priest's prayers continued. Eventually the sacrificial animal was brought forward, blessed again, and lifted by two staff members over the motor of our main office car. With a few swift strokes of the knife, its throat was cut, and as the animal stopped moving, its nearly headless carcass bled profusely onto the engine. Eventually, flowers and the goat's blood would be offered for all the vehicles.

My roiling stomach told me that this was different than seeing an instant decapitation from the viewing stand. This little goat bled to death as I watched. I had to look away, take deep breaths, and battle silently with my confused reactions. My only nightmare-like memory of an animal being killed was watching my grandfather decapitate a chicken when I was about five years old—and the sight of its headless body hopping around the yard, blood spurting, came back to me in scary dreams for a long time afterward.

At the same time, I recognized a respect for the animal that was part of this ceremony, and that the goat would be a source of meat for this community. *Them, maybe, but not me*, I thought, remembering my first evening in the villages struggling to politely consume meat from a goat I'd just befriended. Even so, I knew it would be hypocritical of me as a meat-eater to demean the entire practice. Both the office *pujah* and the public event that I'd witnessed were, in fact, more humane ways of slaughtering animals than most of the abattoirs at home.

But I also knew that if I made Nepal my home for the rest of my life, I'd never truly understand what I'd seen that day. Dashain was yet another lesson in my experience of the vast range of ways that we in the global village live. Taking life was loathsome, but I partic-ipated in it every time I ate a bite of meat, fish, or fowl. Here, at least, the taking had meaning beyond producing a toothsome meal. How could I argue with that?

Chapter 17
Poison

Returning to Gorkha after showing Sita the big-city sights provided a disquieting look at the still-mysterious world that was her home.

Corinne and I traveled back together on a blindingly sunny day. The peace of the trail, after Kathmandu's hullabaloo, was church-like, inspiring. Ferris-wheel *pings* were still in operation from the holiday, so we stopped to play on one and take pictures. Our first sight of the river when we reached Khaireni was disappointing—it looked at least hip-high, still too dangerous to cross on foot, which meant a one-hour detour to the bridge. But a few local men lingered near our crossing point, and they walked us each across for a rupee. I felt safe in the protective grip of my helper, though we'd heard of a porter recently being swept away in unexpectedly swift current.

Then up the famous Cheppetar Hill. A slog, but in the shade of late afternoon it was more of a tiresome chore than the torture I remembered from the first time. The route was so familiar I had the very pleasant sense that I was heading home. The lush green millet fields, the houses, even the people we passed looked soft, natural, welcoming after the relative squalor and crowded streets of Kathmandu. As we approached the Gorkha house, our neighbors were full of cheerful greetings, the kids more energetic than ever with their incessant namastes.

My sense of tranquility lingered after we arrived, despite a zig-zagging flurry of activity as we paid off the numerous porters who'd come with us, unpacked their *dokos*, and organized the supplies they'd carried. After dinner I sank onto clean sheets in my little bed and listened to a new Bob Dylan tape, under the shadowy beams of a Coleman lantern. Because we would work for the coming week in the area just around the Gorkha office/house, there would be no need for overnight treks for a while. I could stay home!

The next afternoon, any illusion that I was living in a peaceful world dissolved in a moment.

Corinne and I stood at the office door while the teams came in to drop off their supplies after finishing work. Gannu, our diminutive but feisty cook-housekeeper, stood in her usual bright-blue apron watching the activity from the kitchen doorway.

As Sita walked in, one look at her told me there was a problem. Her face was filled with worry, anger, disgust—expressions I'd never seen from her before.

"Sita, namaste. How was your day?" I asked her quietly, with a frown of concern. The silence in the room was electric. No one spoke at first, and the other staff who had filed in behind her looked around at each other uneasily.

Sita glared over at Gannu with a look of pure revulsion. Suddenly, eyes shooting fiery arrows, Gannu began shrieking invectives at her. In a moment, the two of them were shouting at each other in what I could only assume was some long-standing feud.

Accusations were volleyed back and forth so rapidly I could barely understand a word, but their mutual fury was clear. One word repeated several times was "*bik*," which meant poison. Corinne and I looked at each other in total dismay. *What on earth was happening?*

"What's going on with you two? Please stop shouting!" Corinne pleaded, moving to a position between the two women. The battle of words slowed, but without any sign of a truce. I could only stand by, dumbfounded, trying to understand what could have caused such violent animosity between these two otherwise reasonable people. Whatever it was seemed deadly serious.

Corinne finally determined that separating the two women was the best short-term maneuver. She went with Gannu back into the kitchen, and I retired to the porch with Sita, along with Sushila and Bhim Raj, the team members remaining, to get the story. Gathered around on the cushioned chairs, Sushila and I held hands with Sita, who was on the verge of tears. Bhim Raj related the tale, his usual grin replaced by a somber frown.

The problem had begun some weeks back, when Sita came to the office with a friend and asked Gannu to make them both a cup of tea. Gannu had refused, saying that the Memsaabs weren't there, and they needed to authorize her making tea for someone not on the team. Sita was annoyed and left in a huff with her friend.

Shortly afterward, Gannu came down with facial shingles, with a lot of pain and a drooping cheek on one side. She consulted Dr. K. C. and then went to a *jhaakri*, who discerned that she'd recently had an argument with someone. That planted a seed of suspicion: Gannu became convinced that the shingles was the result of Sita's evildoing, that she had invoked an evil spirit. Soon all the neighbors knew the story of the accusations, and the resulting furor.

Then it got worse. Friends of Sita's heard about the ruckus and told Sita to be careful, as Gannu was angry and could be planning to poison her. Before long that rumor was all over town. Sita's parents heard the story and were afraid for their daughter's life. Sita was so angry she couldn't tolerate even the sight of Gannu. That afternoon, for the first time, the suspicions and the anger on both sides had all burst out.

I knew something about conflict resolution, but nothing had prepared me for this kind of clash. Sushila and I took some time calming Sita, reassuring her that we'd talk to Gannu, that it was certainly all a big mistake, and she'd be fine. With her face a study in sadness and her shoulders slumped deeply into her blue sari uniform, Sita talked about how worried she'd been, and how angry at Gannu for the false accusations.

"But you didn't even tell us this was happening!" I scolded Sita, who just shook her head sadly and sighed.

"I didn't want to worry you," she said sadly. "But Gannu is a bad woman. I'll never talk to her again."

I murmured something sympathetic and gave her a hug. They left, Sita's two friends saying they'd accompany her back to her family home.

Corinne came out and sat down with me. She'd gotten Gannu's version of the events, simply a repeat of the charges of malfeasance against Sita. We looked at each other and shook our heads in disbelief.

"So that was it, the old poison story," said Corinne. "Sounds like a Nepali soap opera." She looked down the path at our departing friends. "Poor Sita."

"Yeah, poor Gannu too," I added. We'd weathered several small storms with Gannu, who was impulsive and not the best housekeeper, but never anything like this. "We'll have to have a serious talk with her, but not tonight."

We spent a while going over the other *bik* stories we'd heard, and they were numerous. Though I'd never known of a verified incident, rumors of poisonings were not uncommon. Dr. K. C. had told me that many of the autopsies he was asked to perform were because family members suspected poisoning as the cause of death.

Evil spells. Poisoning. Damn! This sounds more and more like fairy-tale land, I thought. But no Sleeping Beauty here. The poison stories came from frightened people trying to figure out why things happened as they did. It was another reminder of the little I really understood of the undertones of this culture, how it shaped people's perceptions of their world.

The *bik* story seemed gradually to dissipate after the open flare-up at the office, as Gannu's shingles improved. We finished work in Gorkha village, moved on to the next *panchayat*, Taranagar, finished there, and traveled on to Namjung for second round of immunizations. The days were fabulously cool and clear, perfect trekking weather. Brilliant scarlet poinsettas were in full bloom everywhere, lining the trails like small trees. With the rains finished, we more often had glimpses of the Himals toward the north, shining above a distant haze. I found myself wandering down (or up) the trails lost in my thoughts, marveling at the beauty that seemed to enclose me in a protective bubble.

Then we were back in the Gorkha house for the week of Tihar, the Nepali festival of lights. I was anxious to get back and pay a visit to the laboratory at the hospital because of a concern about some intestinal symptoms that had begun to plague me. I dutifully presented a stool specimen at the lab, and the next day the laboratory assistant, Dil Bahadur, paid a personal visit to me at the house. He spotted me basking in the sun, sitting out in our yard on a makeshift bench, as he arrived.

"Memsaab!" he said as he charged through the gate. Dil was a young guy, touchingly enthusiastic about his on-the-job-training in laboratory diagnosis, and he was said to be great at identifying creepy crawlies that lived in the gut. "Namaste! You're just like us now!"

I looked at him curiously, then slowly realized the likely implication of his joyous announcement.

"Okay, so what is it?" I groaned with a sigh.

"You have two! *Ascaris* and *trichuris*!" he said. Two of the more common intestinal parasites. Both were treatable, but the thought made me feel queasy all the same. I'd seen stool samples with the *ascaris* worms apparent, and it was, well, creepy. A great many of the Nepalis we tested had at least two and often more parasites, as the organisms were so likely to contaminate food and water or, in the case of hookworm, the soil.

"Don't look so happy, Dil Bahadur," I admonished. He grinned all the same. "How do you recommend I treat them?"

I knew the treatment, of course, a simple three-day regimen of a widely available antiparasite drug. He concurred and left with a victorious smile as he marched back down the trail.

Because it was the week of the Tihar festival, houses around ours were illuminated every night for the first two or three hours after dark with dozens of oil lamps. Tihar, like all the holidays, has special *pujah* days—one being cow *pujah*, when the cattle were garlanded and painted with symbols, often a huge circle in white on the cow's back. Then there was a brother-sister *pujah*, when girls and women gave their brothers a special *tika*, and the brothers brought gifts.

What I called the "song pujah" day was October 31st. That evening Corinne and I were just finishing dinner, chatting about past Halloweens, when we heard a chorus of giggles and shouts coming from the path just outside our gate. I went onto the porch and saw a group of grade school–age kids huddled near our gate. They looked to be mostly girls, with two boys leading the pack. One carried a local drum, a bamboo cylinder with hide stretched over both ends, suspended by a leather thong around his neck.

Corinne hurried out to join me. At the sight of us, the group shouted enthusiastic namastes almost in unison. One of the girls took a step forward and gave a short speech, interspersed with giggles, about Tihar. After a few stops and starts, they launched into their special Tihar songs, accompanied by the drum. The music was, like much of the Nepali music I'd heard, a series of solo lines (or almost solo, as two girls joined voices for that lead role) followed by an enthusiastic chorus. The girls swayed in a little dance to the cadence of the lilting voices.

We listened with a few calls of appreciation for a while, then passed some rupees to a boy who was carrying a shallow basket for that purpose, already filled with coins and a few bills. The group crooned on, long after the money was given out, finally moving on to the neighboring houses.

"So that was our Nepali Halloween," I noted to Corinne as we went off to bed. "No tricks, just a new kind of treat."

After Tihar, the fall days rushed by, an endless stream of immunizations and clinic days, none the same and yet none different from the others. I saw a lot of malnourished kids, in part because we were in the "hungry season," before the rice was ready to be harvested. Every week there was at least one abscess to drain or another child with serious diarrhea.

One evening as I sat at dinner with the team, I looked up to see a young mother standing in the doorway with a toddler in her arms. Even from a distance I could see that the child she held was breathing very rapidly, making little grunts with each breath. Not a good sign, something that couldn't wait for clinic day.

I made a space for them on the mat beside me and asked one of the porters to bring me the medical bag. Though I had my stethoscope, I didn't need it to determine that the little girl had severe pneumonia. As I was explaining to the mother that her daughter needed an antibiotic injection, I looked up to see a local man standing in the doorway, someone I'd seen near camp earlier in the day. He carried a small clay bowl holding some liquid and looked at the little family with concern.

"*Tapaaiko logne?*" I asked the mother. *Your husband?* She indicated that he was not but offered no explanation of who he was.

I found the injectable long-acting penicillin and gave the child a quick shot in her thigh, with the stranger in the doorway closely observing my every move.

"*Daai, ke ke chhainchha?*" I finally asked him, as I finished instructing the mother how to give penicillin tablets at home. *What do you need?* He smiled and came towards us as if he'd been invited in, squatted down, and hastened to explain his mission. He said was a healer and had been treating the child for her problem, but when his treatments didn't work, he agreed she should come to me for care. I was intrigued.

After thanking him for referring the child and explaining what I'd done, I asked about the treatment he'd used.

He answered with a respectful smile. "Memsaab, I only know one treatment for this problem. We need to ask the spirits to leave this child, ask them very forcefully."

Then he hesitated, as if reluctant to give away a trade secret, so I asked, "And how do you do that?"

"Memsaab, you know that cows are holy to us. I said special prayers while I sprinkled urine from a cow on this sick one. Then next, she should drink a little of it, but I saw she was too sick to drink anything."

"So you helped the mother bring her here," I continued, when he hesitated again. He responded with a Nepali nod.

I took in a deep breath, hesitated just a moment, and explained to both of them that, yes, the little girl needed liquids, but plain water with a little sugar or honey and a tiny bit of salt was the best thing to give for this problem, not his remedy. I provided a few packets of rehydration powder, with instructions for using it.

My first reaction at hearing his proposed treatment had been a horrified mental eye roll. Drinking urine, especially by such a sick child who was already dehydrated, was tantamount to ingesting a low-level poison. But at that same moment I could see this man's sincere desire to be of service. He was trying to solve a problem he didn't understand with the remedies he had at hand—prayer and "holy water." Cows were gods, sacred beings, so they would have healing properties. That I had other information and tools was an advantage, but it didn't indicate better intentions or even more brain power.

I sent them off with good wishes and the sense that I'd once again found out something important about the extraordinary world in which I'd immersed myself. There was so much to absorb, so many different ways to understand the mysteries of this culture.

At the same time, an uncomfortable question lurked: I'm learning so much from living with these lovely Nepali people. But will it be nothing more than interesting memories when I leave Nepal, when I go back to that other world I came from? Will I just leave it all behind?

Chapter 18
Giving Thanks

Then it was November, with cold nights and days that were distinctly chilly when we were out of the sun. I wore one of our bright yellow Foundation jackets most of the time. These were the "uniform" jackets that our New York office had sent in an effort, we assumed, to develop the Foundation "brand" in Gorkha. *How New York*, Corinne and I had both said, rolling our eyes, when they arrived. It was absurd to think that the standard marketing approach of promoting a brand made any sense here at all. These villagers will develop some kind of loyalty to the Foundation based on yellow jackets and duffle bags?

Ever since meeting Fred in Kathmandu, I'd begun to question aspects of what we were doing. I doubted that staff in offices in New York really knew what was going on in Gorkha. Why did they need typed reports on each area we covered, so the porters had to carry a heavy typewriter everywhere we went? It seemed ridiculous. Why couldn't we be authorized to provide a few basic medicines when local people needed them, so I didn't have to do it surreptitiously? Couldn't the program also show the locals that we would help them with the problems that plagued them the most? I was to learn much later that this kind of disconnect between policy managers and field-based staff of health and development organizations was not unusual. It was a lesson I would remember when I was myself a project boss in Seattle for a nonprofit organization working in global health: the challenges of staying in touch with the realities of "the field" when based thousands of miles away.

Fall in Gorkha looked much like the same season at home in Montana—lots of fallen leaves, crops being harvested, and earlier sunsets. The late afternoon light shone obliquely, warmer, and paler than at other times of the year, giving me a feeling of homesickness that was at the same time comforting.

But all was not golden. Efforts in a northern area of one of the northernmost *panchayats* had produced some distressing results: Three children had developed abscesses at the injection sites after the first round of our immunizations. We heard about it from Dr. K. C. after the children had shown up at the Gorkha hospital for treatment. He told us that one of the infections was serious, potentially going into the child's bone. We were horrified. Osteomyelitis, an infection of the bone, was notoriously difficult to cure.

Corinne and I, in a short break together at the Gorkha house, went over and over the problem, distraught at having somehow caused harm to the very children we were trying to help.

"Why do you think it happened?" Corinne asked in an anguished tone as we talked at dinner one evening. "We've never had this before."

I thought back to the unusually dusty conditions of that particular area. *Damn!* Probably a vaccine that was out of refrigeration too long, growing colonies of bad little bugs in secret. I felt sick, realizing that it had happened after a visit from the team that I had led. I wanted to crawl inside my skin and never emerge. How could we ever go back to that area? *Those poor families, who trusted us to help them.*

"Whatever it was, I'm going to talk to Dr. K. C. and find out what we can do now," sighed Corinne. "We'll give them money to cover the antibiotics they're getting, travel back and forth to the hospital, and who knows what else? And we'll have to use up open vials right away or throw them out," she said decidedly. I went off to bed that night with an uneasy heart, dreaming of miserable, crying children and angry mothers.

It wasn't only the plight of the individual kids I worried about. Bigger concerns nagged at the back of my mind. If what we're doing can lead to this kind of a bad result, is it the right thing to be doing? Are the diseases that we're immunizing against the biggest problem for these children? Maybe we should instead be doing something to improve care at those badly staffed health posts scattered around the district. We'd done nothing to improve the system that people had to depend on.

My questions, unanswered at the time, would stay with me through my entire career. Years later I would accept the reality that my work in Nepal was, alas, in the category of "well-meaning" efforts without significant long-term benefit. When our program finished, the Nepali health care system was just as limited in its reach into the district as it had been when we started. But ours was at least a relatively low-budget operation. I would eventually see massive amounts of money poured into some of the poorest countries in the world that would leave, similarly, few long-term benefits. And for a similar reason: They bypassed the national system, those most accountable for improving health and living conditions.

But that day I didn't understand the bigger picture and could only troubleshoot the immediate problem. Despite our fears, the second rounds of immunizations in the troubled area went well. The children with abscesses recovered. In addition, because cash was a scarce commodity, the offer of financial compensation to the families was very well received.

"Even that's sad, isn't it?" I wrote in a note to Corinne after we had gone back out with our individual teams, in one of the many messages we sent back and forth via our trusty runner. "Here we do something terrible to their kids, and they're just grateful when we give them money to compensate!" But it was an incredible relief to hear that the children were responding to treatment, at least those we knew about. I set off in a lighter mood to the final area of that trek.

We arrived late in the afternoon, after an arduous up-and-down nine-hour hike. The porters pitched the tents next to a school and we found a small lean-to for use as a kitchen/dining room. The village leader, a tall and elegant-looking silver-haired man, came by almost immediately to greet us.

"Welcome to Arbung," he said with a deep namaste. "You know we have a big celebration here tonight—I hope you can join us," he added.

I steeled myself to respond appreciatively to the invitation. Local leaders were important to the success of our immunization work, and we tried very hard to show our appreciation. But today, yet another *jatra* or festival . . . I thought not. In the fall there seemed to be one every week and, although they were interesting at first, the sameness began to wear on me. I was exhausted, as usual, and my introverted self yearned for solitude. *I really need a couple of hours to myself,* I thought, *whether it's the best thing for the project or not.*

"Thank you so much, sir," I replied, hoping I sounded a bit weak. "I would love to go, but I'm feeling a little sick right now. If I'm better later, I will certainly come."

He smiled in assent. In a place where there was a lot of sickness, it was unfortunate but unavoidable that people would sometimes be laid up during important events. It occurred to me that any kind of fake "calling in sick" was probably very unusual in these villages. People valued their health too much to pretend they were ill when they weren't.

Krishna, who had met us in Arbung, was standing by. He heard the invitation and urged me to go. "I think you will like it—this *jatra* is something like your Thanksgiving," he said. But the thought of that holiday triggered a pang of sadness. Though both were harvest festivals, there the similarities disappeared. One was a comforting memory of family gatherings and very specific meals, the other a mysterious blend of religious rituals, food, and music that I understood would never be mine.

Most of the staff left after dinner to attend the event. *Nope, guess I'm not going to be well enough to go out tonight,* I thought, anticipating my quiet evening alone. Stepping into the big moss-green tent I shared with Sita on this trip, I lit a kerosene lantern and settled into writing letters home and thinking about the holiday season that was about to begin in America. The next day would be the American Thanksgiving, but I'd have no special meal. Because this was our last stop on the three-week trek, the fresh vegetable supply had waned, leaving us with yet another simple meal of *dal bhat.*

I lay back on my sleeping bag and fantasized about my favorite parts of the Thanksgiving meal. I loved the turkey, the stuffing, the gravy on mashed potatoes, the cranberry sauce. And yes, the pumpkin pie, my all-time favorite dessert. I thought about last year's holiday, when my parents and half a dozen friends had joined me in my San Francisco apartment for the whole feast. The delectable smells of the roast turkey were still warming the kitchen the next day, along with the realization of the blessings that came from being loved, being accepted. I'd had no idea then that I'd spend my next Thanksgiving eve holed up in a tent, exhausted after a nine-hour trek. But with no other Americans around to understand the celebration the next day, as well as nothing to celebrate it with, there didn't seem to be any point in lamenting my lonely holiday.

The next morning Sita and I set out early for our immunization site. The day was chilly, with dense green bushes lining the path that were wet with morning dew and brushed against us as we passed.

We found most of the kids we needed to immunize and were on our way back to camp by early afternoon. After only a short time on the return trip, I looked down and gave a gasp. There were at least a dozen tiny, slim worm-like creatures clinging to my lower legs above my tennis shoes. Leeches.

"Sita—look! *Jugaas!*" I squealed. "Not again! Do you have them too?"

"Just a few, I think," she said, lifting her sari slightly to peer at her own legs. Sita was still trekking in flip-flops so she was able to see the extent of the damage right away.

"Why do you have so few?" I wailed. "Look at me—I'm going to be a mess!"

Sita reassured me that she would help me remove the offending creatures. As we charged along for another hour or so to camp, I indulged in a few minutes of woe-is-me complaints to myself. *Good lord,* I lamented. *Now this?* Among the most disgusting critters we had to deal with—fleas, flies, bedbugs, mosquitoes—leeches were the creepiest. In addition to the dozen or more that I could see on my legs, I knew there would be many more inside my tennis shoes and socks. They were little magicians, with their ability to work their way down onto my feet, even as far as my toes, before I even noticed them. Small as they were, they needed to be removed carefully, using salt or a match to get them to loosen their attachment before pulling them off. I knew to do it right this time. My last bout with leeches had left me with a few bites that became infected and took a long time to heal.

We were within sight of camp when I heard a familiar sound coming from behind us, a loud bird call.

As we looked around, Sita burst into giggles. "Look! It's Dennis!"

Indeed, it was Dennis, a young American volunteer who had been working at the Gorkha house to develop a functioning shower and solar heating system. I turned back and even from a distance could recognize his sly grin, tousled blonde hair, and lanky build. He gave another bird whistle.

"Dennis! What the heck are you doing here?" I called out to him.

Pulling closer to us, he gave a big innocent-looking smile and said, "What kind of a greeting is that? I'm here for the Thanksgiving feast, of course. What didya think?"

"Mmmm," I said. "Sorry 'bout that, but we're fresh out of turkey and stuffing. Are you sure you came to the right place?"

Dennis just smiled, and we continued on to camp. He went straight into the cooking hut, and within moments I heard whoops of laughter from the staff. What Dennis lacked in language skills he always made up for in his obvious goodwill and slapstick sense of humor.

Sita and I strategized briefly about getting rid of my leeches, choosing the salt approach. I went into the tent and sank onto my sleeping bag, propping my legs up on the edge of a box of reports, and looked at them curiously. Around some of the leeches I could see bits of blood seeping onto my skin, but now I felt more apathetic than agitated. *I wonder why this doesn't bother me more,* I mused. *Maybe leeches just make sense when everything else around me comes from the Middle Ages.*

Sita came in with a piece of rock salt she had gotten from Bhim Raj and knelt down beside me. She went to work with a little frown of fierce determination, rubbing each tiny creature with salt and then picking it off. She was focused, efficient, dropping each one onto a leaf-bowl that would be incinerated in the cooking fire. After pulling off the last one, she quickly swabbed alcohol on the tiny red spots that were left from the leech bites.

"Thank you, Sita!" I said, and gave her a little hug. Hugs weren't really a Nepali thing, but Sita seemed to understand where it came from.

Once again I marveled at our good fortune in finding someone like Sita to work and live with us. She was such a loyal friend and support, always there to take care of me, whether it was keeping curious onlookers at bay, helping remote village women understand my

Nepali, or picking off leeches. At times I felt that she was my live-in sister, and I was safe if Sita was around.

I jumped up, ready to join the food preparation and hoping Dennis had brought something special. As we made our way into the makeshift kitchen, I heard another voice I knew well. Calling out from behind us came a cheerful, "Hello, girls!"

I whirled around. "Corinne!" I called out in astonishment, rushing back down the trail to give her a hug. Corinne's smiling face was always a welcome sight, but today I was ecstatic to see her. "Are you here for Thanksgiving too? I had no idea you were coming. Dennis is here!"

"Honey, we decided you didn't need to spend your first Thanksgiving in Nepal all by your lonesome!" Corinne replied. "Come see what we have to eat. It's going to be great."

We spent the next couple of hours pulling together a delightful facsimile of a Thanksgiving dinner. Though there was no turkey, Dennis had transported a small canned ham from Kathmandu.

"Is there going to be enough ham for everyone?" someone asked. Clearly not, and here some kind of meat was what differentiated a "feast" from a simple meal.

Corinne responded, "Bhim Raj, can you get a chicken? Everyone needs meat—it's Thanksgiving!" Then, turning to me, "And look—we're going to have the absolutely essential vegetable dish, a green bean casserole!" She smiled and triumphantly pulled two packages of freeze-dried beans out of her backpack along with an envelope of dried mushroom soup mix. "Look at this! What else do we need? We'll use *dalmut* for the topping," she sang, referring to the local crunchy snack made from fried lentils.

The rest of the meal came together from items Corinne and Dennis had brought from the office. For candied sweet potatoes we had a local kind of yam, boiled and mixed with honey. A can of cranberry sauce emerged, a little miracle from another place and time. Easy additions were mashed potatoes and, of course, rice. And then—the pièce de résistance: pumpkin pudding—local pumpkin cooked with milk, eggs, and sugar like a pie, but without the crust.

Finally, the food was ready. The porters looked at all the new dishes curiously, delighted to know about this American festival. Noticing that the light seemed dimmer than it should be, I looked up to see that both windows and the door were filled with fascinated spectators from the village. Their heads were packed into every square inch of available space. I could hear the speculation as they tried to figure out what we were eating for this strange American feast. *Old dried meat from a metal box? Oh, but see, they have rice too, like us. Don't they eat dal? What's that white stuff? Not potatoes!*

"*Haamro Amerkani* Dashain!" I beamed out to the onlookers, saying it was the American equivalent of the big Nepali harvest festival. As we began eating, the audience continued to block out most of the dying evening light. *How fitting!* I thought. Now it was the Nepalis who were trying to figure out our strange holiday food and rituals, instead of the other way around.

Krishna had acquired a bottle of home-brewed *raksi*. We poured generous amounts into our white enamel cups and held them high, toasting to the health of the children in Arbung, each other, and our future success with the program.

Looking around at the group, chatting and joking between appreciative comments and bites, I felt an immense gratitude. After months of festivals that I wanted to enjoy but really didn't understand, we were celebrating one of my own. I reflected that this was the essential Thanksgiving: being with people I care about. The *raksi* and the event brought on a warm, expansive feeling of total contentment. Though we didn't have the classic Thanksgiving meal, what we had was the perfect holiday.

At that moment I was truly grateful to be just where I was, in an amazing place, different from anywhere I'd ever known. Was I learning to accept what Nepal had to offer, in spite of my doubts, my questions, and all the annoyances? Among countless Thanksgiving Day events since then, nearly all slip by unrecalled from one year to the next. This one is embedded in my memory as the best ever, the surprise Thanksgiving in Arbung.

Chapter 19

Tigers, Spirits, and Holy Cows

The following week as we arrived in Arughat and were setting up camp, I overheard an animated discussion between Bhim Raj and an unfamiliar voice. I poked my head out of my tent with an inquiring gaze. Bhim Raj looked over at me and said excitedly, "Mary Anne Didi, *aajah ko baato ma baagh thiyo!*" *There was a tiger on the trail where we passed today!*

"Really! Right where we were?" I asked, astonished. Tigers were well-known dangers in parts of India, but said to be very rare in this area. All the same, we'd heard stories about a man-eating tiger in Borlang a few months prior, so it seemed possible. "How did they know it was a tiger? Did someone see it?"

"No, but it killed a woman who was out cutting feed for her buffalo, in middle of the afternoon. She was partly eaten, on her neck and face," he said, softening his voice to acknowledge the tragedy.

My stomach turned in revulsion as I pictured a woman's ghastly half-face, bloody, bone and muscle exposed. "That's awful!" was all I could reply.

Just then a scene from that afternoon flashed into my mind when I'd been separated from the team. I'd taken a brief detour to get a picture of the Himals from a fabulous viewpoint that I remembered from a past trip. Clustered at one point on the trail was a group of serious-faced villagers, milling around with worried looks that focused on an older man who stood in their midst. It seemed that someone had died, but their discussions were so intense I didn't stop to try to converse with them. Hearing the details later, I realized that I'd probably witnessed the aftermath of the fatal attack on that unsuspecting village woman.

This was something new. In all my travels in Gorkha, I was nearly always with the team, but even during a few side trips on my own, I'd never once felt unsafe. I suddenly wondered what other perils I might have unknowingly escaped. I knew of a development volunteer who was mysteriously murdered several years back. Other possible dangers probably lurked, like loose rocks that could propel me over a cliff to my doom. Or a deadly tropical disease with no cure.

But any of those scenarios seemed unlikely, something my mother back home would worry about, not realistic threats. In fact, I couldn't imagine my team letting any harm come to me, or to any of us. Certainly, I didn't worry about being eaten by a tiger. *But for that poor woman it was the ultimate risk,* I thought. *And a horrific death.*

I was on my last trek before the Christmas break, and we were back in the areas of higher elevation. Though the cool air was great for trekking, the trails to get to our sites were killers, with steep ups and downs, hour after hour. And the farther north we got, the more *jungali* the villages were. Jungle-y. I loved that word—a perfect Nepali term for wild and independent, referring to people as well as places. Now I would think of Arughat whenever I heard that expression.

Despite possible tiger encounters, I found myself more calmly accepting of the constant activity and commotion than I'd ever been. The villagers certainly were *jungali*, suspicious and needing a lot of admonitions and explanations before they would allow their kids to be stuck with needles. But I was mostly unperturbed, sailing through the days with a smile and an occasional *"Ke garne?"* The impending holiday break clearly had buoyed my spirits.

Clinic patients still came and still brought surprises, not so much for their specific problems, but for what the encounters taught me. One day a rather elderly man arrived with a huge gash in his leg that was several days old and infected. I asked how he got the injury.

"It was our cow, Memsaab," he admitted. "She's done it twice before. Her horns are really sharp."

"Twice before?" I asked, puzzled. "Why do you keep her? She may do it again, and this is a bad injury. Next time it could be worse."

"Oh, Memsaab, it's a problem. But our cows are gods to us, so we can't do anything to them. And if I sold her, she'd just injure someone else. Sometimes I'm just not careful enough. What to do?"

What to do, indeed. I sent him off with antibiotics and admonitions to wash his wound carefully the next time the god-animal impaled him.

Holy cows weren't the only beings causing illness or injury. That same day, I had another encounter that surprised me, even though I should have known better by then. We were finishing up a ward, but because too few children were coming, we were making visits to individual houses where the officials had told us we would find small children.

I was directed to the simple, well-kept home of a family with a small daughter about three years old. She'd had the first DPT shot, but hadn't come to us that day for her second one. I sat down with both parents on straw mats on their porch to talk.

"We need to give your little girl her second immunization," I said to the father, after a few opening pleasantries. "Can we do that now?"

"Oh no, we didn't bring her today because she's been vomiting since last night," he replied. "And she had a fever."

I whipped out my packets of oral rehydration powder, useful for either diarrhea or recovery from a stretch of vomiting.

"Oh, that's too bad," I said, looking sympathetically at the little girl on her mother's lap, who clung tightly and eyed me suspiciously. "But I have some medicine that she can take as soon as she stops vomiting, plus something for her fever if it comes back. And we can still give her the immunization."

The child's father smiled graciously. "Oh, she's not sick with a disease," he said. "We're doing a *pujah* because she's under the spell of a spirit. We can't give her any medicine until the *pujah* is over, or she would die."

I could almost see my brain, maybe my whole head, doing an about-face: once again, thinking I saw a medical issue and faced with a totally different perception of the problem. The condition was caused by a supernatural force, so instead of medicine they would have a religious ceremony. How could I argue with that?

The little girl's father added that the child had acted strangely and fallen down just before vomiting, making me think of a seizure. If that had happened, it was perhaps due to the fever. He seemed an educated man, very calm and rational about his child's situation. Seizures, I knew, were considered a serious business of the spirits, and I couldn't urge him to do anything that he believed would endanger the child further.

This man's conviction was another reminder for me of that basic Nepali premise: The first step in dealing with a health problem is to know its cause. If it's spiritual, all the medicine in the world won't help. By then I'd heard many other stories about spirits in Nepal, their powers, their antics, and realized that this spirit world was an everyday reality for nearly everyone I met in Gorkha.

That evening in my tent, in the quiet time after dinner, I let my mind rove around the world that they saw. It was a landscape alive with invisible beings that held power over so much of their lives: their health, their luck, the crops, and the weather. I realized that, at some remote place in my psyche, I could see the spirits too, looking a bit like Saint Anthony, to whom we prayed when something was lost, or Saint Christopher, who could safeguard travelers. Except there were many more spirits here in Nepal, and they weren't all helpful. Some were quite dangerous. This spirit world was complicated, so it was all the more important to understand and respect.

That night, I wrote in my journal:

Maybe . . . maybe there really are some strange spirits running around over here. There is, at the upper left-hand corner of my mind, a faint question. . . .

Because we were working in more isolated areas of the district, the team was the object of particular interest whenever we arrived in a new village. All of us, foreigners or not, were outsiders and thus worthy of attention. Some evenings, the porters would borrow a local drum and set up a dance party for the local young people. On other days the team would just sit around after dinner and chat, the porters teasing each other as well as the vaccinators and me.

As I continued to be more and more in sync with the team, Bhim Raj had special fun bringing up risqué topics. He'd been delighted to hear about Corinne's recent field visit from her Kathmandu-based boyfriend, Michael, who had brought his own tent to share with Corinne.

"So, Corinne Didi has to rest a lot more these days, eh?" he chortled to the group one evening, his toothy grin betraying a double meaning. He used the term *arum garne*, simply meaning to rest, but with an obvious insinuation about her and Michael sleeping in a tent together.

"Oh, yes, sometimes now she's very tired," commented another, to raucous laughter. Most of the team had met Michael at one time or another and were fond of him, pleased that he could chat with them in their language.

"But Mary Anne Didi, don't you ever want to rest like Corinne does?" continued Bhim Raj, again to an appreciative response. He was always ready to push discussions a bit further than anyone else on the team. "We need to find you someone to rest with."

"No, no, I'm always too tired for that kind of resting," I replied, happy to join in with the banter.

I thought about the topic later that evening as I settled into my sleeping bag. Who would have imagined when I was in such an active social mode in San Francisco, only a few months ago, that I soon would be content to lead the single life? Joking about it in a foreign language? Could it be that I didn't need a man to define my importance? Since college there had always been someone, my husband, then boyfriends, interesting people who in some way defined me. I had none of that now. I was encountering a new world, facing challenges I'd never dreamed of—on my own. I smiled contentedly that night as sleep took me away.

Discussions with the team sometimes took a more serious tone. One day as Sita and Sushila and I were waiting at a *chautara* for women to bring their little ones to be immunized, Sita asked about my religion.

"Mary Anne Didi, are you a Christian?" she asked. I'd noticed that Sita was more interested in learning about the world outside Gorkha since her trip to Kathmandu.

A difficult question. Raised Catholic, but not actively practicing any religion, I waffled.

"Yes, my family is Catholic, which is one kind of Christian," I answered. "But when I left home, I stopped the Catholic practices. Like going to the temple." Better than trying to explain Mass, confession, communion, the whole works.

"But you believe in Jesus?" she continued. "Who was Jesus? What did he do?" Sushila added a confirming nod, indicating she was interested in learning as well.

"Well, many, many years ago . . ." I began, aware that it sounded like a fairy tale, and tried in my still-not-fluent-enough Nepali to explain the man, his followers, his theology, and his death. "Christians also believe that he came back from being dead, and now he is the main

God they pray to." Since the three incarnations of the Hindu god were rather like the Christian trinity, the Father, Son, and Holy Spirit explanation wasn't so difficult.

I realized as I went more deeply into the conversation that this thing called religion was another way that this "family" in Nepal mirrored my Catholic family in Montana, as obviously different as they were when seeing only the particulars. They were believers, devout people, accepting very complex beliefs that were not so much irrational as simply outside of that whole realm of logic and rationality. The images, the practices, the ideas were meaningful because they were held in common, shared with a community of believers. And even though I was an outsider to both systems, I was comfortable with them. It was my beloved mother I saw when I watched a devout woman in private moments of worship, at a little flower-strewn statue of some favored god.

Our discussion turned to the parallels they could see between their lives and mine. Parents wanted so much for their children to maintain the old traditions, but growing up sometimes meant leaving the parental ways behind. Prejudice was in the conversation too. We talked about the caste system, my uneasiness with it.

Sita commented, "I know you don't like our caste system, Mary Anne Didi, but isn't it like when you had African slaves in America?"

Bingo.

"Yes, very true. Slavery was about the worst thing we've ever done in America. Black people are still suffering immensely as a result," I sighed. "Here at least the low-caste people have their families and villages. The slaves didn't have that. Children could be sold away from their parents at any time. We also did the same thing with our Native Americans, making the children go away to special schools away from their families."

Both women gave me looks of astonishment, revulsion. Nothing, absolutely nothing, could be more devastating than taking children from their families. I wanted to say more, but there was no way to explain away the horror that was slavery, or describe the devastation that was still felt in African American and Native American families. I didn't try.

Our conversation ended with a trickle of women coming up with squirming children to be immunized, and we went back to work.

Staff would spend some evenings reading or studying. Sita wanted to learn English, so she often carried simple language booklets around with her. At odd moments I'd see her sitting alone, whispering the foreign words to herself. A few wrote notes to their families at home in the main village.

One evening I was surprised to see two of the porters poring over one of the health education pamphlets the Nepali government provided us. I slowly realized that writing skills had become a status symbol among the men. Those who qualified as a *lekne manche*, meaning able to read and write, were enlisted to help with record-keeping when we had a big crowd of children to vaccinate. They would go out with us as a porter, the bluest of blue-collar, low-status jobs, but then at the site become clerks, registering kids and filling in the immunization cards. I could only imagine the thrill for Mek Bahadur, one of our brightest porters, when he took on that task one afternoon and was addressed by the ward official with the respectful term of "Saab." Mek was determined to move up the scale somehow, and I hoped he could. But in our program there was no career ladder, no matter how dedicated or multitalented a person might be.

Mail came weekly, usually with a welcome letter from Mom and occasional missives from friends. One evening the runner came with fresh vaccines and several letters, which I set upon immediately, delaying my dinner. But after reading them, for no reason I could pinpoint, I felt empty, let down. Though friends had written about their activities and asked polite questions about mine, I could feel that our connections were fraying, loose, unsatisfying.

Words from a close friend seemed to capture it: *This experience is really changing you, isn't it?* he wrote. It was. I could see how it was setting me apart from people with whom I used to share a common path. Was I being torn in some irreversible way from the possibility of returning to the life I once knew? What would be left of the previous me when I went back? I felt my isolation again, but differently from before. Now I wasn't longing for the old life, but wondering if I would ever want it again.

Chapter 20
Helicopter Fantasies

Just before dark I trudged across the hanging bridge over the churning Trisuli River into the noisy, smelly little highway town of Khaireni. I'd thought the Christmas holiday would never come. I would spend the night in a grimy little teahouse too near the road, its only "bed" a straw mat covering a wooden bench and rats or some other unpleasant creature rustling about the walls. But there was an outhouse in the back (no matter how rank the odors wafting from it), a water tap just outside my window (although it dripped noisily much of the night), and blessed privacy, so I felt privileged.

I was about to begin a three-week break from Gorkha to work at the US Embassy Clinic in Kathmandu, filling in for the regular nurse who was on leave. I could stay at her house and, in the process, get a better sense of the lives of the expatriate community in Nepal. Would I want to take a job in the relative luxury of the city when I left Gorkha? This was a chance to answer that question.

The next morning at first light, the traffic began grinding its way into frenzied activity. Massive trucks, decorated with fanciful images of fabled Hindu gods, menaced the highway. People along the roadside (there was nothing resembling a street in Khaireni) looked annoyed, distracted, unfriendly. No part of this motorized Nepal, with its diesel fumes and furious clatter, resembled the villages I'd just left. As I scanned the highway for our Foundation car, I felt oddly intimidated, not sure if I could handle the twentieth century again. But my ride arrived on schedule, and suddenly I was en route to my long-awaited break.

When we arrived in Kathmandu, the driver let me off near the north edge of the city at the bungalow where I'd be staying. I found the hidden key under a flowerpot and let myself in.

Stepping inside, I gazed around and marveled at the luxury that was to be mine. A standard three-bedroom house, it had the aura, to me, of a palace. Though the furniture was uninspired, probably embassy loans, the walls sparkled a clean white, the carpets were plush, and I could feel a warm current of air coming from a vent near the door—the miracle of central heating. A little alcove housed an electric washer and dryer, even though someone came weekly to do the wash. I wandered into the modern, fully equipped kitchen with its sparkling white appliances. *All this for just one person!*

Suddenly I was startled by a noise from one of the bedrooms and stepped back toward the door, ready to flee. Out bounded Zack, a golden retriever I'd met once before. He seemed to remember me, barking briefly, then wagging his tail and licking my hand.

"Oh, sweetie, you miss your lady, don't you!" I said, sitting down on an overstuffed chair to give him a vigorous petting. His silky coat felt like a warm greeting from another world, and I realized he was the first dog I'd touched in the nine months I'd been in Nepal. Village dogs were never pets, never trusted not to snap or bite, and they were always happy to donate their fleas.

A paid helper would be coming to walk Zack twice a day, so I could enjoy his company without the slightest obligation. I was told the housekeeper/cook would preparing rice and buffalo meat for him daily, but I was to check at random times to be sure that was really happening. Though it hadn't been voiced directly, I knew that Nepali cooks were regularly accused of taking their employers' food home for their families.

"You're a lucky guy, Zack," I told him. "You get better food than most of the people in this town!" Zack nodded and licked my hand again. That thought made me uneasy, and I sighed. *I'd better get used to this.*

Kathmandu was a dramatic break from life in Gorkha in virtually every way. I cycled or caught taxis to move around town, walking no farther than from the doorway to the street. I was back to speaking English almost full time. The house wasn't far from restaurants and, for a few days, I gorged on Tibetan dumplings, pizza, and fried chicken. I was back to watching the Nepali people from afar, an uninvolved stranger, again sensing the gaps between their lives and mine.

My work at the embassy clinic was the one reminder of my Gorkha life. On my first morning at work, I chatted with the pleasant young American embassy doctor, who was happy to let me be the initial contact with patients and confer with him for questions.

"I'm wondering about some of the problems I've seen in Gorkha, and I'd love to hear what you think I should do for treatment," I said after a short tour of the small facility, which was on par with anything I'd known in the States.

"Sure, just shoot," he replied.

"OK, I've seen this several times: a healthy-looking person, often a young man, with no other problems, but a big open ulcer on his leg." I indicated a two- or three-inch wound, typically on the calf area. "Sometimes he's had it for weeks. What would that be?" I asked.

He took in a breath and shook his head. "You know, I'm not a tropical medicine guy. I've never seen anything like that here," he said after a brief pause. "So, not sure I can help you on that. What have you tried?"

I said I'd given out a long course of antibiotics, and twice was able to get follow-up on the results. Both of those were successful, reported by grateful, smiling patients.

"Well, sounds like you did the right thing. There's weird stuff out there. But here in Kathmandu we see mostly aches and pains, other chronic conditions."

So I was back to seeing Western health problems. The pace of the clinic was relaxed, with never more than five or six patients in a day, rarely involving anything unexpected. Nearly all the patients were Nepali staff of the embassy, and I could order a full barrage of diagnostic tests, xrays, or drugs for even simple problems—all the luxuries of modern medicine. The contrast between the resources at the clinic and what were available in Gorkha—even to Dr. K. C.— were jarring.

But if I was shocked and a little uneasy with this new role, an expanded social and cultural life made it seem worthwhile. My friend Jane, after finishing her doctoral degree, was back in town, and we had several evenings to chat over dinner. My old San Francisco friend Arnie and his wife included me in an occasional evening at the movies. Most of the Foundation staff were also on a break for the holidays, and I was soon invited to a steady stream of holiday events. I went with Corinne and Michael to a documentary on the migration of the African wildebeest at the home of the cinematographers who made the film. Another evening, we heard a lecture by an anthropologist studying cultural aspects of specific Nepali tribal groups. *Hey, I like this life!* I reflected several times during those first few days.

Other events were simply gatherings of expatriates that appeared to have the primary function of reminding everyone of their common origins: from somewhere else, not Nepal. One Saturday evening, Jane and I went to a small party at the home of an American embassy staff member. I gazed curiously around the living room where a small group sat sipping generous glasses of wine. Except for the tastefully arranged paintings of Nepal's iconic mountains and an array of local baskets, I could have been sitting in a middle-class home anywhere. But this was the first glass of wine I'd had in months, and I relished it. An embassy connection meant access to liquor sales at the embassy exchange; otherwise local beer was the only alcoholic beverage available commercially in the country.

I looked around at the group. All were based in Kathmandu with some international agency, all were white, and all had firm opinions about what needed to be done about the challenges of development in Nepal.

"I've been here long enough that I'm beginning to feel jaded about the prospect of any progress at all," said one man, a clean-cut, young-looking aide to the ambassador. "Seems like one step forward, two steps back, most of the time."

"Really? I thought the new five-year plan was starting to take shape," said another. "Can't do everything at once."

"And there's so much that could be done!" gushed a woman lounging across from me on the floor, whose red hair added to the air of total confidence in her pronouncements. I later learned that she was a wealthy heiress, formerly employed by one of the embassies. "I heard an awful story last week, about a village woman in Jumla who died from appendicitis. Died! And she could have been so easily treated in Kathmandu!"

Others in the group nodded their heads sadly. Getting good surgical care in the rural areas, even the district capitals, was rare indeed. But that was, surely, no surprise to anyone.

"I've been thinking about how the government should have helicopters available when something like that happens," she continued. "I wonder how much that would cost."

I stifled a gasp. *What world was she from?* Bringing the critically ill or injured to Kathmandu via helicopter was a great idea, and in fact that system was already in place. But of course it was only available for exatriates or the very wealthy, people with money in their purses or from their organizations, like the Foundation that employed me.

The image of a helicopter magically swooping down to take me on a five-minute ride to our destination was one of my favorite daydreams as I slogged, sweaty and dog-tired, along the trails in Gorkha. But it was a farfetched fantasy. So was the thought that air-lifting poor villagers off to Kathmandu for medical emergencies was what they needed most. The vast bulk of the rural population often couldn't even get from their home to a functioning clinic for basic care or afford to shell out money for services of questionable quality once they arrived. So many more lives would be saved by a well-run national system of doctors, nurses, and clinics with services that were free and accessible to the villagers.

No one else seemed particularly puzzled by the heiress's pronouncement, so I ventured a reply.

"But there are lots of people in the districts who don't get care for even simple problems—shouldn't we start there?" I asked. "How would the country ever pay for that kind of helicopter service?"

She looked thoughtful and mused about how it should be possible, somehow. Maybe they could establish a special program.

I felt myself slump into the chair, unwilling to give any further attention to such a mad idea. I'd already figured out that "establish a program" was the common development response to challenging problems, which all too often remained intractable despite numerous efforts. They resulted in hopeful-sounding campaigns, like posters advising villagers to "Plan Your Family," which were widespread in rural areas, despite zero availability of modern contraception in many if not most districts.

The conversation drifted off to other subjects, warnings about the anticipated traffic jams for the king's birthday parade coming up, and a new store about to open that would sell frozen buffalo meat. I studied the group, trying to read their thoughts, gauge their responses to what I'd heard. Nothing. What was I missing? I knew that I was relatively ignorant on the sophisticated topic of "development" in Nepal, barely even understanding what the term meant. But was I the only one in the room to think the helicopter idea was, at this point in time, just a ridiculous daydream?

Later, I realized that the woman's wealth and elevated status likely explained the polite reactions of the group. But I had other discussions during my time in Kathmandu that gave me pause about the kind of help that was coming to Nepal from other countries and organizations. How much did the "aid" world understand about the realities of the country's rural areas or the challenges to the national health ministry? I spoke with staff of large agencies who were loathe to live outside Kathmandu, preferring to travel back and forth to a project area daily rather than endure living in primitive village conditions. I talked with others who, even after several years of working in Nepal, had yet to acquire anything but the most rudimentary skills in the Nepali language—rudimentary, as in, "Bring tea, please." I began to doubt the impressions I once had of all the good that was being accomplished by the millions of dollars of foreign aid coming into the country. And I wasn't quite sure I wanted to be part of that system.

I didn't know then that Nepal would struggle for decades to make significant advancements in getting services to the rural areas. But the country would eventually produce a viable national health care system, with maternal care, including contraception, widely available. US Peace Corps volunteers and others who had lived in rural areas eventually found their way into the aid agencies, bringing that valuable experience to new programs. Roads were built and, over time, most district centers had modern hospitals and qualified staff. Mortality rates improved dramatically as well. For example, by 2016, deaths of women due to childbearing were said to be less than half of the rates of 1998.

Yet in Nepal, as in most countries even now, average numbers still don't tell the stories of the hardships of life in remote areas. When I look at figures for national-level data, I imagine the women I'd met who lived far from any clinic or health worker, and who suffered—or watched their children suffer and sometimes die—at home.

Despite my reservations about the expatriate role, as Christmas drew nearer, the holiday spirit overtook me. Santa Clauses were everywhere! I should have guessed. . . . Nepalis love their holidays, so adding another one or two was an irresistible opportunity to celebrate.

Christmas Eve was a quiet dinner with friends. Afterward, though I'd not been to church around the Christmas holiday since leaving college, I went alone on an impulse to midnight Mass at St. Mary's church. The piety of so many Nepalis took me back to my childhood and the years of our faithful attendance at Mass every Sunday, and I felt a need to connect with those nearly forgotten rituals. The service felt intimate, deeply meaningful. This was my tradition, just as surely as *pujah*s and *tika*s were the culture here.

The New Year brought something truly new: a change in country director. Our new boss, Stella, was a charming, trim woman in her forties. She had worked in Kathmandu for the Foundation for many years previously and was returning from sick leave. Having an initially good impression of her, I decided that the time had come to give my notice. I asked for a meeting and cycled to her office one afternoon after leaving the clinic.

"Mary Anne, I'm so happy to have a chance to get to know you a little," she began. "I understand you're doing great work out there in Gorkha. Corinne is very happy to have you on the team."

My heart sank an inch or two. *It'll be so much harder if she's really nice*, I worried. On the edge of a straight-backed chair facing her, I was anxious about how to proceed. My previous attempts at announcing my potential early departure with the New York boss hadn't gone so well.

"Thank you. But I have something difficult to tell you, and I guess I might as well go ahead and say it," I plunged on.

"Oh, I know, you're having a hard time with the thought of spending the rest of your Foundation time in Gorkha," she said with a kindly smile. "I can understand that. It's tough out there."

I was stunned. *She knew! She maybe even sympathized, at least a little.*

"Yeah, that's about it," I mumbled.

"Well, maybe you've heard that we hope to have government approval for the video project in the next couple of months. And with our video volunteers gone, we need someone to get that project going." She paused. "Would you be interested in working out the last six months of your contract doing that? It's very different from what you're doing now, but I think you could handle it," she added.

I had a momentary lurch of hope, then shook my head doubtfully. "That would be fabulous. But, to be honest, I know absolutely nothing about video technology, and not even much about health education except what we're doing in Gorkha."

"No, of course not, I know that," she replied. "But you don't have to be the expert. You'd be working with two people in the Ministry of Health who'll be in charge of the project, help them get it started, find out where and how they can be trained. The Ministry is interested in seeing if video might work here."

Now I was more than stunned. After months of agonizing deliberation about what to do, how to justify breaking my contract, an ethical escape hatch had just materialized. It would be a chance to start out the right way, working alongside Nepalis instead of trying to "lead" them. We talked for another few minutes about what the project would entail, and with very little hesitation I told her I'd be delighted to take it on.

In the space of those few minutes, an invisible load had just been catapulted off my shoulders. I found myself shaking my head, over and over, wondering why I'd been so worried, when a simple solution was all it took. Like the deus ex machina in ancient Greeks plays—I had my god from a machine. Her name was Stella.

After the holiday celebrations died down, I still had another week to enjoy the city. But by then, ironically, the novelty of living in Kathmandu society had diminished like a cheap Christmas toy. I wasn't particularly anxious to get back to the drudgery of long days on the trail, but now I had to deal with seeing myself in the role of an office-based "advisor." Would I become just another Kathmandu expatriate?

Chapter 21
The Birth of an Untouchable

After the holiday break, the remaining January days whirled by, moving quickly into February. The landscape began to look parched, and hills that had been lush green were turning amber, the terraces brown and bare. Many of the villagers were occupied hauling fodder for their animals from points far from their homes. Every day on the trail we met young people so burdened with masses of dried grass and tender branches that I thought of them as walking haystacks.

The whole project seemed to have suddenly changed. A light was shining brightly ahead of me, a respectable way to finish up my work. Though it still didn't seem quite real, there was a new lightness to my days. Then Corinne's time with the Foundation was up, and after a farewell party at the Gorkha house, she headed back to Kathmandu. I couldn't quite imagine being without her cheerful energy and enthusiasm, and the notes we sent each other incessantly about the work, our tribulations, and joys. Two nurses, one British and one from Ireland, were coming soon as replacements for Corinne and, later, for me. We were hiring a new vaccinator too, Sundaree, an enthusiastic young woman who even spoke some English.

We'd also acquired another advance man, Captain Limbu, a retired Gurhka army officer. He was from one of the ethnic groups that had served with legendary courage in special regiments of the

British army, beginning in the early 1800s. Captain had excellent English and a military bearing, with a solid build and a square, East Asian–featured face. He seemed a good addition to the team.

One evening, as I returned to camp after a full afternoon vaccinating, a young man approached us on the trail and asked politely if I could come with him to check on his wife. When I asked what her problem was, he replied that she was in labor with their first child and it was taking "very long."

"How long has it been?" I asked.

"*Hijo baata*," he replied. *Since yesterday.* "It's been a long time. We live very close, just five minutes away." With that he pointed, with a jut of his chin, to a small settlement nearby that did indeed look only a short distance off. I agreed to go with him, stopping first at camp to pick up the delivery kit.

We quickly arrived at a simple house in the middle of a small hamlet that Captain had told me was a village of Kamis, one of Nepal's untouchable castes. The young man I'd seen on the trail ushered me inside, then quickly disappeared.

It was still bright daylight outside, but I stepped into a room that was, at first, dark as a cave. It emanated a pervasive gloom that only such shadowy, spongy rust-colored walls could produce, absorbing as they did most of the light from two flickering oil lamps. I could faintly see a young woman crouched in the far corner, moaning in pain, with an older woman by her side. I paused to let my eyes adjust to the dimness, then introduced myself. I learned that the laboring woman was called Sani. The older woman, her mother, told me with a drawn, worried look that the contractions were getting closer together. She looked at me intently, as if deciding whether or not I was a safe confidant.

"Can I examine her, please?" I asked the mother, and she nodded in assent, apparently satisfied with my offer of help. Sani herself barely registered that I was in the room. I helped her lie back on the straw mat and within a few minutes determined that the baby was in the right position, with a strong heartbeat, and the young mother-to-be was almost fully dilated. But this was her first pregnancy, so the delivery could take a while longer. I reassured the family that the baby would come before long and said I'd return soon.

Two hours later, dinner finished, I sauntered back to Sani's house to check on her progress. I'd expected to see the young woman in the comforting care of her mother, but what I found instead was an eerie, other-worldly scene that would stay with me long after I left Nepal.

Stepping into the still-dark room, I could see Sani squatting in the middle of the mud-pack floor. She was leaning against her mother, who supported her on one side, with another older woman holding her up on the other. Behind them in a slightly elevated area was an assembly of five or six ancient-looking village women, some sitting on the floor and others standing in a kind of crouch. Beside the women flickered a low-burning open fire that occasionally illuminated their faces in ghostly flashes. All were focused on Sani.

In the semidarkness I couldn't see anyone clearly, but the role of the characters in this drama was obvious very quickly. The women barked out commands at Sani, first one, then a chorus with the same admonitions—like a flock of harpies, I thought, unkindly.

When she saw me approaching, Sani's mother called out plaintively, "*Sakena, sakena.*" *She can't.* The group of women immediately echoed her words, adding a string of concerns: *The head won't come. She won't push. She has to . . .* and on and on, in an excited babble. The faces of the women in that faint shadowy light were haunting. I could see that they were engaged in a ritual that everyone understood. But for me it bordered on surreal and was oddly frightening. I had been transported to a kind of netherworld, one that seemed more dream than reality.

But I was there for a real-world reason. Putting down my bag, I took out a flashlight and knelt beside Sani to check on her progress.

She was fully dressed, and even in her extreme state so modest she would barely let me lift her plaid lungi for a view of what was happening. When I finally succeeded, I saw at once that the baby's head was crowning, and the delivery was imminent.

"*Tik chha, tauko niskinchha,*" I said to Sani's mother. *It's fine, the head is coming.* I reached for my bag to get the plastic sheet to avoid her having to deliver the baby onto the mud- and dung-packed floor.

"*Tauko niskinchha,*" the women chanted in response and began urging Sani in a frenzy to push, push, push. I wanted the women to cease their commands, to let Sani rest before her last major effort, but realized I was powerless to affect the momentum of this ancient rite. As I laid the plastic sheet out onto the floor and began to help Sani move onto it, there was a sudden gush of something bulky from under her skirt. I lifted the edge and, sure enough, there she was, a full-term little baby girl.

I gently lifted the infant onto the plastic, horrified at the sight of her lying on such an unclean spot and at the same time exhilarated at the beauty of this new little life. She opened her eyes briefly, astounded, I was sure, at the sights around her. Then she let out a lusty cry, that riveting moment that lifts the heart of any participant in a birth. I looked around at the room with a jubilant smile, elated—and saw that I was the only person in the room with the slightest interest in the newborn. The women were instead intent on accomplishing their next task, getting Sani's placenta delivered.

The chorus began again. "Push, push, push," they chanted. Then, from one, "Make yourself vomit, like this," demonstrating the finger-down-the-throat technique for inducing a gag reflex. Sani was mostly oblivious to their commands, but after a few minutes made a feeble effort at putting her fingers in her mouth. She heaved weakly, looking around in exhaustion.

Before long the placenta, too, slithered out from under her skirt with a rush of blood. I checked with my flashlight to be sure it was intact, since if any pieces were left behind, it could lead to bleeding, infection, or both. It was all there.

The next task for the group was supervising the tying and cutting of the umbilical cord. I had a heavy silk string ready for the occasion, but Sani's mother was concerned that it was too thin and brought me a substitute. I nodded and pulled out my sterile scissors, explaining how important it was to keep the cord area very clean. The women all nodded their heads in agreement, "Very clean, very clean."

Suddenly, looking with concern at my scissors, one of the women blurted, "Do you cut it all off? Or let it fall off later?" I assured her that, of course, the remaining cord had to fall off after it dried up. Murmurs of relief. They had, naturally, no way of knowing what strange birth customs this foreign woman might practice.

"Sani has to do it," her mother said, referring to cutting and tying the cord. Though I wanted to support their traditional practices, poor Sani was so exhausted she could barely keep from toppling over.

"She's very tired, isn't she?" I said.

"Yes, but she has to do it. We can help," Sani's mother replied.

Compromising, I tied off the cord at the level they indicated, gave Sani the scissors, and helped her cut it. The placenta went into a large leaf-bowl that was placed beside us for that purpose. It would be disposed of ritually, according to the tradition of the area, whatever that might be.

I wondered if the ritual was over. No, cleansing was the next step. As birth in the Nepali culture is considered highly polluting, one woman had added a few sticks of wood to the fire and placed a pan of water over the three large stones that served as a grate. Sani changed her blood-stained lungi for a fresh one, still following step-by-step commands from the gallery. Then she was directed to bathe the newborn by pouring the warm water over her and smoothing the blood off the baby with her hands. The commands continued.

"Use this cloth. No, not that one, that's to wrap her in. Don't you know anything? And not too much water the first time," they went on, unrelenting. Then, "Now, take out a breast and feed her. You have to do it right away or she won't have a good appetite later."

"She won't take the breast? Here, do it like this," said one ancient woman, who whipped out her own saggy breast and showed Sani how to milk it. "Like this. Hold her closer."

Finally, the baby made a few nuzzling attempts at nursing, and murmurs of approval emanated from the women. Satisfied that their mission had been accomplished, one by one they harrumphed, made a few parting comments, and took their leave. I checked the young woman for excessive bleeding and also left, promising I'd return in the morning to visit the new mother. Sani's mother helped her daughter onto a straw mat in a corner where she could, finally, rest with her new baby.

On the short walk back to the camp, I marveled at how different this delivery had been from the previous one I'd attended in Aru Pokhari. There, the family had given over management of the delivery to Corinne and me. Here, I was a small player in some bigger system. I puzzled over possible explanations. Sani's had been essentially a normal delivery, where Maili's had been dangerously prolonged. But here I was in a Kami village. Was this intense ritual related to their caste identity? The earlier family had been Brahmins, the highest and priestly caste, said by some to be hapless in dealing with earthly matters. Who knew? It was another of the many mysteries of this culture that I'd never really grasp.

When I returned to the house the next morning to check on Sani, she was sitting outside against the wall of the house with her sleeping newborn, her own mother by her side. They greeted me, and Sani held the baby up to show me her fresh, beautiful little face.

I reached down and touched Sani's shoulder. "What a perfect little girl you have," I told her. She smiled and gazed adoringly at her firstborn.

I took out my camera with a questioning look and received a proud smile in response. Snapping a picture of the lovely trio, I wondered what the future would hold for this child. Surely she deserved the best that life could offer, but what was in store for her?

Even though caste discrimination had been officially outlawed in Nepal since the early 1960s, years before my time in Gorkha, that cultural reality had never come close to disappearing. The lowly status of Kami "outcastes" like her would be a central element of the social system of Nepal far into the future. She wouldn't be allowed to enter temples, eat at common gatherings or with higher-caste people, drink from public water sources, or marry a higher-caste man. Her surname would always identify her as being of lowly status. Even if she had a basic education, her future would include few employment possibilities, worse poverty compared to most other Nepalis, and virtually no representation in government or other power circles. It was hard to imagine a more complete description of discrimination against a group that constituted some 15 percent of the country's population.

Kamis and other untouchables were so far down the status ladder that they weren't actually seen as being within the caste system. Once again, I wondered how "outcaste" Nepalis could accept their status with so little apparent resistance. I knew about the ideas of karma, dharma, and transmigration of souls. Maybe those concepts helped individuals build a picture of the world that would allow them to accept their place in it. But they were also excuses for a really ugly system of hereditary inequality, one that turned people socially into something less than truly human.

Centuries of living under the thumb of one group or another seemed to doom many Nepalis to acceptance of situations that were, to my foreign eye, atrocious, uncivilized, insufferable. In addition to the indignities of caste, reminders of women's absolute subservience to their husbands disturbed me deeply, reflected in practices

I tried to forget about but couldn't. Wealth was another enormous imbalance. Even within Gorkha, many of the village leaders were prosperous beyond their evident earning power, with multiple wives and homes. Corruption was said to be rampant at all levels. It seemed that inequality was burned into the Nepali psyche, a permanent part of the culture.

During my first few months in the field, I felt overwhelmed trying to grasp the meanings of the ancient ideas and practices I came across and understand the depth of their hold on the population. I'd mentally railed against the Nepali acceptance of whatever happens as being "just the way it is." Then, eventually, the confusing array of customs and traditions began to be somewhat comprehensible. I could see a rationale behind many of the customs around personal behavior, traditional healing practices, beliefs in a powerful spirit world, and religious efforts to cope with unseen forces. But caste was different. Each time I encountered the unmovable reality of how the lowest castes were viewed by otherwise reasonable, kind people—my friends!—I found myself screaming inwardly that this system was both disgusting and cruel.

I understood that nothing I could do in my few short months there as a privileged outsider would have any effect on making it a fairer system, or on the lives of people who were anointed at birth as being unworthy. So I rarely voiced my opinions to my Nepali counterparts, instead trying to find short-term remedies to any caste-related issues I had to deal with. Should I have been more forthright about the injustice that I felt so deeply? That troubling question followed me to bed that night.

Entrenched systems of inequality are of course not limited to caste distinctions. Later, when I was in graduate school studying the reasons that some groups of people have better health than others, I came to realize the profound effects of the kind of caste system that dominated my own country. Health in the US was so clearly related to social and economic class; richer white people did better than non-whites and the less well-off. The Black population was particularly disadvantaged, whatever their wealth or education. In Nepal, inequality meant caste, but in the "advanced" nation that I had returned to, the results of racial and class inequality were and still are blindingly evident, every bit as destructive as caste in Nepal. A quote from the economist Amartya Sen stays with me: "I believe that virtually all the problems in the world come from inequality of one kind or another."

Chapter 22

Mountain Vistas

What an impressive team! I surveyed the ten porters, four vaccinators, and two new nurses, Jean and Ann, who would be taking over the program. In addition to Captain Limbu, we had a new interpreter/advance man from Kathmandu, Shakiya. All were gathered outside the Gorkha office with me. "*Tayaari bhayo?*" I belted out, mimicking Captain Limbu's military style. *Are we ready?*

"*Hunchha!*" was the rousing reply. *We are!* The porters set out in the lead, passing through the gate and down the trail from our office.

After months of being cancelled and rescheduled for various reasons—weather, illness, vacations—I was setting out with both teams combined on this longest, most challenging route to date. This was to be my last trek, a final, bittersweet farewell to my year in the field. We were headed to Barpak, the highest and farthest north *panchayat* of the area we covered. Although not more than eight or nine thousand feet in elevation, we would be in much greater proximity to the Himals, the mighty Himalayas.

Filing out with the team, I smiled encouragingly at the new nurses, Jean and Ann, seeing that their faces reflected more anxiety than enthusiasm. *Understandable,* I thought. Both were around my age and were enthusiastic about learning everything they could from my experience. One was British, one Irish, with the expected look of bewilderment in the early stages of adapting to this crazy life, learning the language, and getting accustomed to the strenuous life of daily mountain hiking. Fortunately, they seemed to be developing a close relationship. This was to be their last trek before they would take over leading the teams themselves. I wondered what was going on in their minds.

What was going on in mine a year ago? Looking back at those first few weeks in Gorkha, I saw a very different person from who I was today, this confident leader charging down the path. Overwhelmed with the strangeness of every aspect of my new life, I'd been uncertain then if I had the skills and endurance to survive the isolation and challenges that each day was bound to bring. But what had been bizarre and mysterious then was everyday-comfortable now, and I was eager to take on this one last challenge. Whatever the angst or uncertainty I'd felt a year ago, this day was pure elation. Despite the usual early morning chaos of organizing the tents, sleeping bags, cooking gear, food, immunization equipment, and dozens of smaller items, it felt like the opening day of a celebration.

Krishna had gone ahead the previous week. He sent back with a local traveler a series of warnings about what we might encounter, scrawled on a smudged piece of notebook paper. "The trails are steep and very narrow," he wrote. "Some of them might be dangerous for porters because our regular *dokos* could make them lose their balance and tumble down the mountainside."

He reported that he'd slipped off the trail at one point himself and had to be hauled back up by a group of local men. He also found that many of the people spoke only local languages and didn't understand Nepali. The houses were so spread out that getting help from the local officials would be difficult. In many of the villages no one was literate, so we wouldn't always have lists of children who needed to be vaccinated. Finally, there were dire warnings that tigers roamed the jungle at night, and ferocious dogs randomly attacked travelers.

In spite of (or was it because of?) the possible danger, the prospect of this final challenging trip was alluring. I was confident that the staff could handle any of those challenges and more. They were my team, and I knew them, trusted them. We were safe together.

"Mary Anne Didi, *khusi hunuhunchha*?" asked Bhim Raj with his usual grin, looking back at me as we jounced down the trail that led out of town. *Are you happy?* He and I had talked about this trek for months, and he was as energized about it as I was. I smiled back, with a sideways Nepali nod.

Of course I was happy. Since my first look at the Rocky Mountains on a Montana family trip when I was ten years old, mountain scenery had captivated me. The first sight of those distant, shining mountains on the horizon as we neared Billings was startling, electrifying, a dramatic contrast with our familiar prairie landscape. Until then my only view of mountains had been a solitary painting of a majestic, rosy-hued peak that had hung on the wall of our country school, right by my desk. I'd gazed at it, drawn by the lure of its unfamiliar beauty. The exciting world of the future, my future, seemed to beckon from that enchanting image.

For two days we plodded north along the Darandi Khola, the river that bisected the district, with steady ups and downs that weren't especially arduous. It was April, so neither the heat nor rains of summer had set in. The heavens were cool and cloudless, the sun dropping a peaceful, warm mantle on the rocky trail and hills or valleys on either side of us. At random moments I found myself looking around at the team, trying to fathom the reality that I would never again be in this special place, or with these people I had grown to know so well. Most of the time, though, leaving felt like a distant concept. Reality was now, the muffled crunch of seventeen pairs of feet on the rocky trail, the screech of bird calls, and the occasional bantering voices of porters or vaccinators. *Maybe I've learned to just be here today, and not worry about tomorrow,* I mused. *So Nepali of me.*

On the second afternoon, I looked off to the right and saw an elegant flowering tree, with pale pink blossoms shaped like tulips. As I stopped to admire it, I noticed two of the porters rushing off the trail to gather up the blooms.

"Bhim Raj, what do they want those flowers for?" I turned around to ask the cook, who was coming up the trail behind me.

He answered with a sly smile. "You'll see, you'll see," was all he would say.

That night we were served curried *phool,* or flower, for dinner, a supplement to the usual rice and lentils. Bhim Raj grinned at me as I tentatively lifted the aromatic blossom to my mouth. "*Meetoh*?" he asked. *Is it good?*

"*Meetoh*!" I replied. I was tempted to add, "Tastes like chicken," but refrained, knowing the joke would fall flat. It actually tasted like any bland vegetable that had been perked up with curry spices.

On the third day our climb steepened for several hours as we approached our destination, Barpak village. The trail became rockier, the vegetation more sparse. As the trail grew steeper yet, I began to tire.

"Are we almost there?" I asked in English, to no one in particular. No answer.

The team was used to just smiling at my plaintive pleas toward the end of a trek. The worst thing they could do, they had found, was to say, "Yes, we're almost there," when another couple of hours remained. Silence and a sympathetic grin was a better option.

And then, as we rounded one last rise, I stopped, stunned: The sparkling sunlit crags of the Himalayas loomed up before us. Like a movie panorama, gigantic snow-covered mountains rose on three sides, towering over a deep valley of tree-covered hills that sloped down from the base of the highest peaks. They were taller, bigger, more majestic than any photo could ever show. The sight was even more breathtaking than I'd expected.

Our work up to then had been in the "middle hills" of central Nepal, ranging from four to five thousand feet in elevation. They would be called mountains in most other countries, but not here, where they were flanked by the highest peaks in the world. From some earlier villages, we had a distant view of the Himals, but nothing approached the grandeur of this sight. The scale of everything seemed to change in the presence of these giants.

The real mountains, I thought. *I'm finally here.* I was in the midst of that future I'd wanted, and it was more exhilarating than I could have anticipated. If there was such a thing as a perfect moment, this had to be it.

Straight ahead, hovering above the valley, was a treeless plateau with a settlement of small houses in its center, the village of Barpak. We sped up along the trail and approached the village, its homes quite unlike the charming thatched-roof cottages of the lower areas. This settlement of Gurungs and Ghales, groups that dominated these higher altitudes, instead consisted of boxy houses very closely spaced in a compact village. Some were even attached in squared-off rows, with nearly flat slate roofs and well-framed doors and windows. The impression was rather stark—except for their view of the most spectacular mountain scenery in the world.

We peered into the distance, looking for the center of the village, our usual rendezvous point. Finally, I spied the familiar figure of Krishna coming along the trail to greet us. He waved and flashed his signature white-toothed smile.

"Mary Anne Didi, welcome! How was the trip?" he asked, barely pausing for my reply. "Ahh, you will be so happy to see your home for tonight," he said, with eyebrows raised as if a special prize awaited us. He greeted the rest of the team and led us to an open area at the edge of the village, indicating that it was to be our camping spot for the night. A small stone building sat in the center.

I glanced around. "Thanks, Krishna. Looks very nice. . . ." I muttered, with a shrug of mild disappointment. It looked exactly like our other campgrounds: a flat enough area to put up several tents, a large room that could be used for cooking and for the porters to sleep in. But Krishna gave another grin and nodded at me to follow him. With Sita and the other vaccinators trailing along, he led us down a short path away from the encampment. The trail led to a one-story, slate-roofed stone house surrounded by a fence of the same stone and built up against a rock outcropping. *We'll stay in a regular house here?* I wondered, curious now.

"This is your palace for the next four days!" Krishna announced dramatically. We went through the gate, and he pulled out a set of huge old-fashioned keys and unlocked the rough wooden door. I stepped over the sill, suddenly energized after the long day's trek.

Amazing. Clearly this was not a normal Nepali cottage. Though the air inside was chilly and musty from weeks of being closed up, the light from the ample windows illuminated a scene that nearly took my breath away: wooden living room furniture with thick, comfortable-looking cushions! A stone fireplace! By now Jean, Ann, and the three women vaccinators had arrived. We raced around the house inspecting the details: real beds in two bedrooms, with cushy foam mattresses. A kerosene burner and wood-burning stove, with an oven, in a small kitchen. A sink with (drum roll!) running water, piped in fresh and cold from a spring. An outhouse was attached along the side of the main structure, another luxury.

"This house belonged to a British man who lived in Barpak for several years, working on a foreign aid project," Krishna explained, pleased with our excitement. "When he left, he said the house could be used for housing visitors, and we are of course special guests!" He smiled again proudly, and then left us to our settling in.

A Brit, of course. Nothing else would explain the presence of such relative luxury in a setting where every available resource was used judiciously, for essential needs.

"Okay, girls, this is the life we were meant to live!" I joked and sank into a chair, a little amused by my response. Who would imagine that sleeping in a normal house would be so exciting? But it was a kind of fantasy that I had never dared have in all the past months of living in a tent, moving from village to village. At the time, the irony escaped me: I was in one of the most spectacular mountain environments in the world, yet almost as thrilled by having a familiar-style home for a few nights as by my proximity to the mountains. Maybe this was training for the return to a "normal life" after Nepal.

We parceled out the beds among the six of us. Sita and I had one of the double beds, with a deep foam mattress covered with a quilt and Indian-print bedspread. It was a bit dusty, but as inviting as if it had been the smoothest satin. We grinned at each other as we threw our packs onto the floor beside the bed.

"Watch this, Sita!" I said, and with a running jump bounced onto the bed. She looked startled, and I realized she had probably never before had a mattress thick and soft enough to jump on.

In celebration we had an early dinner that evening and hurried to our beds—real beds, not mats. The kerosene lamp gave just enough light to make bedtime reading possible, so Sita poured over her English language notebook as she often did, and I scribbled notes in my journal about this glorious day.

Putting her book down, Sita settled under the quilt and squinted over at me with a sad expression.

"What's wrong, Sita?" I queried.

"Mary Anne Didi, this is our last trek together, isn't it?" she responded softly. "Then you'll leave, and we'll never see you again, isn't that right? I don't want you to go, no one does."

I felt a dull mantle of sadness settling over me, reminding me of an impending pain I didn't want to face. "Oh, Sita, my friend," I replied with a deep sigh. "I have to leave. But I'm also very sad thinking about it. I hope you don't forget me—I will never forget you. I won't forget any of this. And Corinne and I will come back to Gorkha to see you, really we will."

I could feel my voice begin to waver, my eyes swell with tears. This was what I didn't want to think about yet. Yes, Corinne and I planned trips back to Gorkha, but a visit could never be the same as this life that I shared so intimately with all the team. She had been my closest support for the past year, a daily figure in my life, my field sister. And I feared it would be many years before I saw her again.

I blew out the lamp and we talked for a while longer, about a new job she hoped to get when this one was finished, about my next few months in Kathmandu. With our last few words barely finished, we both drifted to sleep.

I rose later than intended the next morning, behind the rest of the staff. As I was about to set out for the main camp, I saw Krishna approaching the house, accompanied by a local man.

"Mary Anne Didi, there's someone important you need to meet," he announced, rather breathless, as they arrived. He introduced, first in Nepali, the slight, undistinguished-appearing man who accompanied him. Then he pronounced in English, with a dramatic flair, "This is Manu Ghale, the king of the Ghales."

Ah, the traditional leader of the Ghales.

"*Namaskar*," I greeted him with a deep bow and the more respectful version of the usual namaste greeting. "We're so happy to be here in Barpak. Won't you come in and have some tea?"

He gave a gracious nod and settled with Krishna into the living room chairs, while I bumbled around trying to light the kerosene burner. *Damn!* I thought. *Where is all the staff when I need them?* I eventually got the device lit and joined the men with a tray of tea at a makeshift coffee table.

Manu wore the usual western-style dark pants and white shirt of the more educated men in the area. He had a gentle manner and spoke very softly. "I think you'll see that Barpak is different from other places you've been in Gorkha," he said, as he sipped his tea.

"Many of our men go away to be Ghurka soldiers for the British and send funds home to their families," he said. "When they retire they come back and sink into ways of drinking, playing cards, and idleness. We had very good traditions, but they are changing. We used to all be vegetarian, but now people think they should eat chicken. What to do?" he lamented.

"It's really hard, isn't it?" I replied. "It's the same for us in America. People have to move to the cities to find work, and when they come back, they're very different. Like I will be when I go home," I added with a smile. We chatted for a while longer, and he left with a polite bow.

As exciting as it was to be there, our Barpak results weren't great. Many of the families weren't home, having moved up to their summer mountain pastures with the children. The vaccinators lamented that the trails were steeper and the population more sparse than in other places we'd worked. That meant more time spent walking when house-to-house visits were needed.

Then there was the ice problem. We were so far from the office in central Gorkha that the ice packs sent from there for our vaccine coolers were mostly melted by the time the runner arrived. I talked to the team about a backup plan. After some discussion, we sent a local man in the other direction, up into the mountains, to gather snow and ice from the slopes.

But those hassles were minor annoyances. I woke up each morning reveling in the realization that I was working and living in such close proximity to the mountains. The three massive pinnacles of Himalchuli, nearly twenty-six thousand feet high, were visible all day, rising to the north like a promise of all that could be. I was later to have friends who made an attempt to climb Himalchuli's main peak, unsuccessful because of early snow and avalanches. But even the attempt looked entirely impossible from my vantage point, many thousand feet below.

On our last morning in Barpak, I rose early and looked wistfully around at the comforts of our house. I decided to treat the six of us— the nurses, three vaccinators, and me—to a luxurious alternative to the usual *dal bhat* breakfast: pancakes with honey, fried eggs, and instant coffee. After flipping the last pancake, I sat down at the table for our last meal and smiled proudly at being able to show the three Nepali women a "real American breakfast."

Jean and Ann both made appreciative comments. I looked at the vaccinators.

"So, do you like it?" I grinned expectantly at Sita as she took her first bites. Sita was usually the first of the vaccinators to accept new ideas, always ready to learn new ways.

"Ah, yes, Mary Anne Didi," she assured me. "Very delicious. When do Americans eat this kind of food?" The other vaccinators seemed keenly interested in my response, glancing back and forth between the two of us.

"Well, not every day," I explained. "But in the mornings when we want more than just bread or cereal to eat."

In the brief silence I sensed, rather than saw, a slightly horrified reaction from all three.

"So, not rice?" Sita asked with an undertone of incredulity. "You never eat rice in the morning?" I could see her trying to process this information but not really grasping the reality of it. A rice-free meal was an oxymoron in the Nepali lexicon. I shrugged my shoulders and smiled, realizing once again the vast gap between this world and the one to which I would soon return.

Filling my lungs with the unique buttery pancake scent, I reflected with satisfaction that I was simultaneously both at home and in the glorious mountains of Nepal. But in the very next moment, a pang of sadness struck me from a hidden, painful place. *Don't forget: This is also the end of it.*

Chapter 23

Final Trails

Endless disasters. The day we were to travel from Barpak to Gumda, the freezer packs that arrived from the office the night before were totally melted, and the backup plan of ice carried from the mountain hadn't materialized yet. We waited. When the exhausted villager-porter finally arrived, the cooler was packed with snow rather than ice. I worried that it wouldn't last long enough to keep the vaccines safe, but *ke garne*? Then as we were about to set off, several sick people showed up begging to be examined—a bad headache, a sick two-year-old, a thumb abscess. Some of the porters seemed to be ailing too, maybe from the Barpak water, and sweet-faced Bakta, our youngest and smallest guy, was not well enough to carry a load. Finally, the few local porters we had hired neglected to bring their own *dokos* with them, so there was another delay while some were located. Typical problems for a travel day, though.

Another issue marred the start of the day. Captain Limbu asked to meet with the leadership team in private just before we set off. He said that one of the porters had noticed that a sari he was carrying for a vaccinator was smeared with menstrual blood.

This was a problem. I knew that touching anything related to menstruation was taboo for Nepali men, a part of the culture I found both fascinating and repugnant. The porter who found the sari was horrified. He talked to Captain Limbu, who discussed it with the other porters. They agreed, he said, that to carry the vaccinators' saris was in conflict with Nepali customs, and it should not be required.

"Captain, do you think this is an important problem?" I asked, curious.

"Yes. They are determined that they shouldn't have to do it, and I agree with them," he replied.

"Well, this isn't something we can deal with very effectively just now, partway through a trek, is it? What do you think we should do?" I asked.

"The vaccinators could carry their own saris," he suggested.

I sighed. This sounded like a precedent that I didn't want to set but, unable to come up with any other ideas, I agreed. "Fine, for now. Can you ask the women if they would retrieve their saris from the *dokos* and put them in their daypacks? And let everyone know that this is only for this trek—we will look into it when we're back at the office."

We finally set off around nine, the team separating into two groups. My team would cover the main settlement of Gumda with Sita, Kaliwati, and Shakiya, and the other half of the team would go to Laprak, a smaller village nearer the mountains. The day was clear, with Himalchuli sparkling on the horizon. Once more I felt a mantle of contentment settle over me as we started out on another cool but sunny day.

Our first four hours consisted of a climb up three thousand feet to a ridge overlooking Gumda and the adjoining area, Kerauja. We soon reached a dense section of deciduous forest, almost a jungle, with few signs of agriculture. Around a small bend in the trail, a brilliant wall of rhododendrons rose up before us, full-sized trees with brilliant red or pink blossoms like Christmas ornaments filling their branches. When we stopped for a short rest in the shade on a steep section of trail, Bhim Raj brought me one to taste, assuring me that this particular flower was a delicacy when eaten uncooked. Not exactly delicious, I thought, but maybe the blossoms in a salad would be good. Then I chuckled to myself. *Salad!* When did we ever have one of those out here? Anywhere in Nepal, uncooked food of any kind was an invitation to giardia, amebic dysentery, or some other intestinal disaster.

As we started our descent into Gumda, another four hours on the other side of the ridge, fields of the local food staple, potatoes, were prominent. The other vegetation of interest was marijuana, growing wild and profusely all along the trail.

In one large field, I spied an older woman energetically clearing a heavy growth of the "weed." She was bent over in the hot sun, wearing the maroon velveteen blouse of the Ghale and Gurung women. Half of the small freshly weeded field held healthy-looking potato plants, and the other half was a mass of greenery, more marijuana than potatoes. The woman was muttering to herself, in what I imagined was a string of curses.

"I'm going to stop a minute—I need a picture of this," I called out and pulled my camera out of my daypack, saying to her with a smile, "Namaste, *Aama. Foto kichne?" Take your picture?* She looked up with a frown as the camera clicked and muttered something I didn't understand.

"What did she say, Shakiya?" I asked.

"Oh, just that maybe you want her to die," he replied sweetly. "Some Nepalis think that when their picture is taken, it shortens their lives."

What? How could I have lived here for nearly a year and not known that? I wondered. *Amazing. And I think I'm so involved in this culture!* I gave the woman another smile, this one laced with apology, as we moved on down the trail. *Another example of the more I learn, the less I understand about this place,* I thought.

I suddenly noticed that several of the porters were snickering at my interest in the marijuana plants.

"Shall I get you some, Mary Anne Didi?" chuckled Bhim Raj,

always the first to tease, especially about anything slightly risqué. We all knew that some Nepalis, including the porters, used marijuana moderately but it was formally off-limits for the Americans. Nepal had been known for too long as a haven for hippies in search of cheap drugs, and the government had clamped down on the practice.

"Yes! Can you?" I asked, with a wide-eyed smile and what I hoped was an innocent air.

"*Hunchha, aajah raati!*" he replied with a Nepali rocking nod. *Sure, tonight!* Everyone laughed, and we continued down the trail.

A few hours later we trudged into Gumda village, which was a dirtier and smaller version of Barpak. Children of varying ages, in ragged clothes with smudged faces, roamed the main path. In these mountain villages, water sources could sometimes be a several hours' walk away, so the precious commodity wasn't used regularly for personal hygiene.

The sight of me elicited startled reactions from the kids that might have been a parody of someone watching a Martian spaceship drop off a few passengers. We paused, wondering where to find the health post, where we would camp.

Despite queries from several of us, the children looked puzzled and gave no response. This was also a Ghale village, and clearly none of them spoke Nepali. But eventually two of the older boys figured out what we wanted, indicating that they would take us there. We filed after them on a path that led through barley fields to another smaller settlement. Beyond that was a complex that included the school, village meeting house, and a health post, all made of local stone with rusted, dubious-looking metal roofs. We quickly dropped our gear into the designated area, deserted of staff at this late hour, and set up camp for the night.

I was in luck again: Now that the teams were separated, I had my own tent! I gazed admiringly at the soft blue igloo as one of the porters popped it up in front of me. Although barely wide enough to allow me to lie flat, it was mine! Pitched in a grassy field, it had a startling view of the shining white Himals.

Just as I prepared to slip inside, Shakiya ambled up.

"Nice view, isn't it? That one is Ganesh," he said with a smile, chin pointing to a central massif that jutted up in a perfect right angle, like a children's drawing of a mountain. Ganesh, the elephant-boy god of the Hindus, has his own mountain, and it was spectacular. Around it rose a jumble of smaller peaks, all of them towering over us mightily.

"Ganesh is a holy mountain, you know," Shakiya added. "Because of that we can't climb it, and anyone who tries is doomed to fail, maybe to die in the process."

I frowned at that revelation. "So, Ganesh will kill anyone who tries to enter his territory?" I asked, hoping my tone was properly respectful.

Shakiya laughed. "Oh, it's just something people believe. Because it's holy, they don't want climbers to ruin it."

I nodded in agreement. Whether because of religious beliefs or just a concern for Mother Nature, there is such a thing as sacred.

My time in Nepal had certainly broadened my sense of the divine. Seeing devout women doing a daily *pujah,* worshiping at the small shrines of their favorite Hindu god, was so much like my own mother's Catholic piety that I felt I understood the practice. But Hinduism was not the only spiritual way in Nepal. The shaman, one type of traditional healer, could be from the much older animist world, called on to identify and heal spiritual and sometimes social causes of health problems. In the more mountainous areas like Gumda, many were Buddhists. Muslims were also a small minority in some districts.

Most fascinating to me was the easy cohabitation of combinations of these belief systems without any obvious clash among them. I had never heard of religion-based conflict in Nepal. In Kathmandu, some Hindu shrines were well-known for including images of Buddha among the gods they venerated. I sometimes ruminated on all the religious wars underway elsewhere in the world, and wondered how Nepal had been able to seamlessly meld so many sets of beliefs. Was it because they began with a clear sense of the sanctity within the natural world? Not one god, but many?

I looked out at the stunning scene in front of me. From the end of the field where we were standing was a precipitous drop to a massive valley sheltering the Buri Gandaki River. Kerauja, the third and final area we were slated to cover after Gumda, spread over the steep slopes to the right. It looked pristine, with no visible trails, and with several long, shining waterfall ribbons and a patchwork of deforested areas. It was beautiful, but the thought of Krishna's warnings—steep drop-offs, suspicious villagers, wild dogs—was beginning to make me uneasy. Should we go there, as planned, after Gumda? Was it worth the risk? That would have to be decided soon.

Exhausted but elated at the privacy my tent would provide, I crawled inside for a quick rest before dinner.

By the time I came out, a gaggle of onlookers, mostly women with children in their arms or clinging to their skirts, was posted outside, lying in wait for my appearance. Here, where very few foreigners had ever come, I was even more of a celebrity than in the lower areas. They peered at my clothes, so different from theirs, commenting to each other on every detail of my appearance. The women wore long-sleeved blouses with the usual thick sashes that kept their long skirts in place. Because it was colder, many had large woolen wraps around their shoulders or heads. It was a charming group, with their bright, open smiles. They looked at me as if wishing we could be friends.

After a year of regular surveillance by these understandably interested folk, I had found a curious peace with being the subject of endless observation. Of course they found a foreigner fascinating, and naturally they marveled at how different I looked. At last it felt okay. Though most spoke only their own language, I did my best to offer a few pleasantries, wanting to provide a friendly glimpse of what the outside world was like.

The next morning as the team finished breakfast, a young man emerged from the nearby health post and turned towards our encampment. He was tall and thin, with longish hair, wearing the black trousers and sparkling white shirt that identified him as someone who was not a native of the area.

He introduced himself with a shy smile.

"Namaste, Didi. I am Sailendra, health assistant for this post. We are most grateful for your coming here. May I know your name?" His English was very good, and he spoke so formally that I understood this was an important moment for him.

I introduced myself and the other staff nearby, and explained why we were in Gumda. When I told him of my health care background, he looked elated.

"If you have time, perhaps I can show you some of my more difficult patients in their homes," he suggested.

"Yes! I could go this morning," I replied, as it was my official day to stay in camp. I was overjoyed at the idea of discussing his patients and what he was able to do for them at this remote outpost. We arranged to meet after the immunization teams had been dispatched to their sites.

That day in Gumda was an education for me in many ways. Sailendra had finished a one-year program in Kathmandu to become what in the US we would call a physician's assistant—except there were no physicians to assist within many days' walk away. After finishing the program, he was placed on his own in this remote rural area, far from his home in another part of the country. He had minimal supplies and equipment and essentially no technical support or backup. Sailendra was of the Newar ethnic group and didn't speak the Ghale language, so he had to do much of his work with an interpreter. Yet for all those constraints, this young man was remarkably idealistic, capable, and clearly dedicated to doing the best he could with what he had.

We set out for the home of a two-year-old boy he feared had pneumonia as a complication of measles. We trudged out of the village a short way, rounding a small hill behind the main settlement. As we drew nearer the house, I began to hear eerie howling sounds echo down the trail toward us, growing louder as we approached. I gave Sailendra an anxious look, and he turned to me with an expression of pain that I will never forget.

"Oh no. We are too late," he said softly, looking despairingly at the source of the sounds. Sailendra knew only too well that we were hearing the distinctive wail made by women when someone had died. More than just a death, in this case that of a child who he thought might have been saved with a few doses of penicillin. But health post supplies of that drug, like many others, had been depleted months before. The child's parents could not afford the expense of the full day's walk to the nearest store where drugs were available.

We approached the house and spoke with two older men sitting outside, relatives of the child, who told us we that were too late, even if we had medicine. I did in fact have injectable penicillin in our supplies, and had I arrived a day or two earlier it might have helped the boy.

We moved into the shadows of the low-slung house and stepped inside, where I could see an elderly woman sitting on a mat, holding the body of a small child, pale and still, in her arms. She was half-singing, half-crying an ancient sound of mourning, rocking him gently and fondling his face, arms, and legs. It was a painful sight, almost too difficult to witness. I took in a deep breath, fighting back tears of empathy, an immense effort to keep my composure in the face of this tragic scene.

"There's the boy's mother," whispered Sailendra, pointing with his chin to a younger woman weeping quietly next to the grandmother.

In her arms was an older child who was apparently also suffering from measles. Various other adults and children milled about the shadows of the room. Dust motes floated in the small beacon of sunlight coming through one small window.

We went up to the two women and both bowed our heads to them in sympathy in a deep namaste.

"*Kasto dukhha, Aama,*" I said to the grandmother, and then bowed respectfully to the mother. *So much pain.* She looked up with the saddest of eyes and nodded her acknowledgement. We stepped back out of the house.

"This is what's the hardest for me," sighed Sailendra, as we started back down the path. "I could do so much more if I had more medicines, and maybe a microscope to help with diagnoses. But in Kathmandu no one remembers that we're even here; we're too far away. And everything we get runs out long before it should."

I'd grieved with others who had lost loved ones, and it would never be easy. But here I wanted to do more than mourn. I wanted understand what was behind these tragedies, rather than focus on the end results. *Life isn't fair for so many people*, I thought for the thousandth time. Wanting to make it a bit fairer was a worthwhile aim, even though I had no idea how to do that.

We saw other patients that day with complicated health issues, and I was impressed with Sailendra's assessments of the problems. He had iron supplements for a pregnant woman who was severely anemic, and I contributed a diuretic for a man whose feet were grossly swollen from a heart problem. We saw a seriously ill older woman whose lung problems and enlarged heart were so far advanced that she could probably not have been treated adequately in any medical system. He presented each case to me with a clear description of what he had diagnosed and the treatments he gave.

As we went from house to house, Sailendra plied me with questions about what I thought, what else he might have tried or could try. I realized that he had been in this job for months, with no opportunity to talk to another medical person about his work and no guidance with difficult problems. If a patient was beyond his help, the nearest hospital and doctor were a two or three days' walk away—with no guarantee that adequate care would be available there either.

Sailendra's was a story I would remember for the rest of my working days, repeated over and over in many other countries and settings. Health budgets of many of the poorer countries, small to begin with, are typically spent on higher-level hospital care in capital cities. Rural areas are left with the bare rudiments of a health care system, and rural health workers are paid a pittance, barely enough to meet basic needs. In many countries the pattern was a legacy of European colonial rule, where the colonizers would provide enough health services to keep the urban native workers from dying en masse, ignoring the rural peasants.

I wondered at first how Nepal fit that pattern, as it had never been colonized by an outside power. But after the massacre of the royal family in 1846, the despotic Rana family rule was as tyrannical and exploitive as that of the colonial Europeans. The Ranas suppressed any signs of discontent and exerted absolute power over an impoverished country, enriching themselves. The allure of "modern" western medicine also led to funding expensive hospitals, rather than more basic primary care. Although my time in Gorkha was nearly thirty years after the Rana family had been unseated, neglect of services for the rural poor was still extreme.

After spending time with Sailendra, I could see ever more clearly that the problems he faced were not something he could ever solve. He was competent and dedicated, but in a system so unresponsive, his hands were tied. I'd heard talk in Kathmandu about the "laziness" of health staff—for example, not showing up for regular clinic hours. "Corruption," asking for small amounts of money from patients to provide what should be free services, was also said to be a big problem.

But what would I do in those conditions? I wondered. It would be hard to continue to care if I worked for starvation wages, and those in power were indifferent to my problems, many corrupt themselves.

For the next two days in Gumda I was back on the puncture-the-babies-and-make-them-cry detail, and touched base with Sailendra briefly in the evenings. On the morning of the fourth day, we packed up for a relatively short journey to meet up with the other team.

Sailendra came by to see us off, with a slightly mournful air. "Go well," he said with the standard Nepali farewell. "*Maya na maarnuos.*" *Don't forget us.* We namaste'd, and I promised to say a good word for him with health officials in Kathmandu if the opportunity ever came up. But I knew it wouldn't.

As our crew of porters and vaccinators was about to set off down the trail in the early morning light, I spied a small band of women approaching us from the village. As they grew nearer, I was puzzled by what looked like flowers cradled in their arms. Everyone stopped, gazing curiously at the unexpected sight. Then three smiling women stepped forward and presented Sita, Kaliwati, and me with arrays of vibrant pink and red roses, the stems wrapped in huge thick leaves to protect us from the thorns. The women had no words for us, just shy smiles and nods.

There were whoops of delight from the porters when they realized that the flowers were for us. Roses. I couldn't have been more incredulous. Here, deep in the high hills of Nepal, we were being honored with the most elegant of blossoms. I was deeply touched, trying not to be teary from the delightful surprise. *I don't even know how to tell them in their language how lovely they are*, I thought wistfully. We thanked them as best we could, with our own smiles and nods and deep namastes, hoping they understood our gratitude, and set off down the trail.

These women may live too far from a water source to keep themselves and their families washed, I thought, *but they understand beauty, and they are the most gracious people I've encountered yet.*

Many years later, the homes, families, and livelihoods of these remarkable people would be devastated by a massive earthquake that would flatten most of the houses and kill thousands. Gumda and Barpak were at the epicenter of the 2015 disaster. A road approaching the area that was built in the 1990s collapsed in the quake, cutting off most routes of support. What remained were the same steep rocky trails we had traveled, accessed only by porters carrying on their backs relief supplies of food, tarps for shelter, and medical necessities to the stricken population.

As I sat in my comfortable home in Seattle, attached to the computer screen in disbelief by images of the disaster, I remembered the roses, the women, and their smiles that day. It was a bittersweet memory.

Chapter 24

Complications

I picked my way carefully along the steep trail that wound down the mountain from Gumda, looking back anxiously at the porters periodically to see how they were navigating the narrow path. The spectacular Ganesh Himal loomed off to the north. Ahead and far below I could see where the Maacha Khola and Buri Gandaki rivers joined at Khorla Besi, the village where we were to meet the other half of the team coming from their work in Laprak. After four hours of a steady descent, the trail dropped off to follow a cliff-like face, where it became steeper, rockier, more difficult to traverse than anywhere we'd been.

I was used to well-worn pathways, wide enough for travelers to pass each other without difficulty, but this one was different. The steep, smooth slope had little vegetation, and the gravelly path was often not more than eight inches wide. I glanced furtively to one side, noting the few hundred feet I would fall if I slipped off the trail, and thought about how much trickier it must be for the porters, with their heavy, bulky *dokos*. *Nope, better not think about that,* I decided and went back to a single-minded focus on putting my feet solidly in the right places in front of me.

Eventually the trail flattened out onto grassy clearings and terraced barley fields, with the low roar of the river telling us it was nearby. Suddenly there was color again: new wildflowers, a tree with a profusion of orchid-like blossoms with a heavenly scent. Butterflies of several colors zigzagged around me, birdsongs rose from all sides, and the spicy aroma of a pine forest and unseen flowers filled the air. The few houses that we saw had the familiar steep thatched roofs instead of flat slate. I felt unexpectedly exhilarated at being back in territory I recognized.

"Was that the last of those awful trails?" I asked Bhim Raj, who was filing along just ahead of me.

"*Sambhav chha*," he replied. *Could be.* His voice was flat, with a tone that didn't sound like Bhim Raj. A few minutes later, at a rest stop under a huge banyan tree, I asked him to step aside with me. He reluctantly lowered his *doko* onto the stone wall of the *chautara* and followed me a short distance from the group. We stopped in the shade of some smaller trees, and I looked at him inquiringly.

"*Daai, ke bhayo? Samasya bhayo?*" I asked. *What's happening? Is there a problem?*

Shoulders slumped, looking down, he muttered that everything was fine. But his eyes told me something else. Nepalis are not known for talking in depth about their feelings, but I decided to press him for at least a hint of what was eating him.

"Bhim Raj! *Bhannos na. Kina khusi chhaina?*" I asked. *Tell me! Why are you unhappy?*

Bhim Raj sighed and began a sad litany of his concerns. Corinne had left, and now I was leaving. He was used to us, felt that we were his friends, and that we liked his work. But he'd spent time with the new nurses and they were angry with him all the time, not happy with their job, not friendly, and he was worried about future treks with them. His dejected look made me think of a whipped dog, past the point of expecting anything good to happen. As we spoke, two other porters eased up to us to join the conversation, and echoed Bhim Raj's sentiments.

Seeing my always-sunny pal looking so miserable was a blow to my otherwise upbeat mood. Worse, I couldn't deny what he was saying. These were early days for the new nurses. One was very critical of Bhim Raj—understandably, after seeing him cough over our meals and use a dirty towel to wipe the dishes. Both were unhappy with the food, the conditions, the organization, and the work in general. I wasn't actually surprised, thinking it a fairly normal response to being dropped into this unusual life that I'd been living for the past year. But at the same time, I wanted badly for them to be kind to these dear people whom I'd grown to love. It felt very much like my own family was being attacked, and I struggled to find the best response.

"I know. This is a difficult job for anyone, and they're having a hard time now. I think after a while it will get better. We just have to take it slowly until then," I offered. "It will be hard for everyone for a while."

They all gave half-hearted Nepali nods and, all of us looking downcast, we made our way back to the group to set off again. Despite my assurances, I had no idea what the atmosphere would be like after I left, but later I was to learn that both nurses ended up being very positive about the program and well accepted by staff.

And I'd learned by then that walking improves almost everything. Within an hour I felt more optimistic as I spied the familiar sight of our tents on a small rise. The Laprak team had already arrived and was ready for us. We moved into camp to the welcome aroma of rice boiling and onions and spices frying. There was a flurry of greetings as everyone prepared for the evening meal.

After dinner I gathered with program staff in the big green vaccinators' tent for a full report of their time in Laprak. We sat cross-legged in a circle, the new nurses, vaccinators, and the two advance men. I asked each group for their sense of the trip.

"It was really hard!" said Jean. "We walked forever on those horrid trails and still could hardly find any kids." Ann nodded in agreement. In fact the vaccine coverage results were dismal, hovering around half of what we expected.

"And then this happened," Ann added, pointing to Sundaree who sat with a swollen ankle propped up on a backpack. One of the precious ice packs rested on it, wrapped in a towel. She had slipped on one of the precipitous trails and couldn't walk without sharp pain.

All agreed it had been unusually difficult: treacherous trails, communication problems with villagers and village leaders, and bad weather, all conspiring against them.

When it was Krishna's turn, he started by saying that he agreed about the difficulties they had encountered. Then he added, "And we had one village that was impossible. The people were very uncooperative. The minute we explained what we were there for, all the mothers just up and disappeared without a word. They scattered like rabbits!" He paused for effect. "So I went to the village leader and asked why the people seemed so afraid of us. He told me that last year a Japanese team had come through to give BCG vaccinations. After they left, all the children got a big sore where they gave the shot, and it lasted a long time. Everyone was worried when that happened," he added, "because no one told them to expect it." He paused.

"Then, six weeks later, disaster struck!" Krishna added dramatically. "A measles epidemic hit the village and sixteen children died. Someone said it was because of the shots they had gotten, and now they're very afraid of any kind of vaccine."

I was horrified. Normally the vaccine we gave to prevent tuberculosis resulted in an infected-looking lesion on the upper arm that later scabs over. It would be very disturbing to parents if that new "sore" was a surprise, and I could only guess the worst imaginings of the families of those children. Even evil spirits, as much as they were feared in this culture, never had as devastating an effect as these flesh and blood foreigners who said they had come to help.

On top of the "black needle" rumor, here was another, just as disturbing. Again I thought about the "we know what's good for you" approach to this rural work. Especially where most people had so

little education, it was hard to resist the attitude: *We have degrees.
We know so much more than these villagers.* But what a mistake. In
the short term, if complications happened, and parents didn't have
the basic information about what we were doing—and what problems could occur—they would of course be distrustful the next time
around. The loss of those precious children meant that families in
that area wouldn't trust any kind of immunization for a long time.
And who could blame them?

But even more importantly—these rural people were grownups!
Even if they needed help to improve the lives of their kids, that didn't
require treating them like they were children or of limited intelligence. I was furious at those unnamed, unseen aid workers who had
blithely gone on their way, never even knowing the distrust and fear
they'd sown.

As other team members had their say about conditions in Laprak,
the vaccinators were mostly silent, nodding in agreement. "Anything
else to add?" I asked, looking pointedly at them. They indicated they
didn't. They were Nepali women, accustomed to letting the men or
the foreigners do the talking.

"Okay, sounds like there were a lot of problems," I said. "Now
there's a decision to make. We're scheduled to go to Kerauja tomorrow, but everyone tells us it will be even harder there. We've heard
that the trails are so narrow we'll probably need special *dokos* for the
porters. Hardly any of the villagers are literate, so there may be no
records of where the children live. They're very suspicious of outsiders, which won't help either. But we're scheduled to go there, and we
have enough supplies to do it. What does everyone think?"

Captain spoke first. "We always hear these rumors, but I don't
think it will be any worse in Kerauja than Laprak. Maybe better. I
think we should go!" He was joined by Krishna and Shakiya in
enthusiasm for continuing with our plan. They sounded cheery, with
a manly energy for forging on.

But both new nurses expressed vigorous disagreement. The team was already exhausted and discouraged, they said, declaring that the effort wouldn't be worth the small benefits. I noted the vaccinators watching with, again, determinedly neutral responses.

It was up to me as team leader to decide, and I hesitated a moment before plunging in.

"Okay, I have to admit I would personally love to finish this trek with a look at someplace that's really different from where we've been. And from here the weather looks like it will be okay. We have the time." I wanted to validate the comments in favor of going on.

"But . . . we'd have to leave someone behind with Sundaree if we decided to go. She can't walk for a while on that ankle. I'm worried that those trails look even worse than those in Gumda and Laprak. And I really can't justify the risk of more injuries, maybe serious ones, given what we know now. So we'll head back tomorrow. Aaru Pokhari is on our way, and we can finish up our last round of vaccinations there."

There was a small shout of approval from the porters, who were peering in through the tent door. Clearly they'd also been worried about the dangers or difficulties of forging on. Walking a steep trail with a small daypack as I did was one thing, but carrying a 70- or 80-pound *doko* on their backs was a much greater challenge on trails that were narrow and steep enough to push them off balance.

We moved slowly out of the tent and started off towards our sleeping areas. "*Ekdum raamro kaam, sabaai-laai,*" I said. *Excellent work, everyone.* "Good night and sleep well," I added in English.

The avid English learners in the group proudly retorted in their sweetly accented tones, "Good nah-eet, Mary Anne Didi!"

The evening air was starting to cool, so I crawled into the tent and zippered the flap shut. I planned to make an entry in my journal, but the writing part of my brain was vacant, non-functioning, so I gave it up. I blew out the lantern and slumped into my sleeping bag. Then the day's events began to race around like a fast-forward movie in my mind. Every detail was there: the women and their roses in Gumda, Bhim Raj's sad face, the long trail out of the mountains, the meeting, and the decision to change our plans.

So much had changed since my first trek to Gorkha village, gasping my way up Cheppetar Hill. Of course I'd gotten into shape physically, able to enjoy even steeper uphill climbs in a way I hadn't thought possible. Many of the mysteries I had first encountered were no longer mysterious. The language was now familiar, and even though I wouldn't call myself fluent, I was proud when I noticed that the dialog in my dreams now was sometimes in Nepali. My team and the people we worked with had provided me with an encyclopedia's worth of impressions about how they lived and saw the world, what they wanted from this earthly existence, what they suffered and why, how they celebrated, what they believed and believed in.

Added to all the new information was a very different me. Since childhood, I'd been a conscientious, compliant person, ready to do what was expected of me. I wasn't a leader, never the one to take chances or forge new paths, simply a good follower. But in Gorkha I'd stumbled into a world that was as foreign to me, as unpredictable, as if I'd landed on the moon. Every day I confronted the need to figure things out, to calculate and make decisions in ways I'd never done before. And—surprise—I saw a more authentic "me" emerging as time went on. I evolved into a more independent, insightful, capable, and determined woman. This new person had the confidence to step into an unknown realm, confront it, and become part of it. As unprepared, naïve, and self-doubting as I'd been when I launched into this new life, my time here had shown me strengths I'd never thought I had. And I really liked the new me.

The next morning Sundaree's ankle was less swollen but still very tender. In a quick discussion with the team we determined that I would stay with her and Ram, one of the porters who was also a good cook, while everyone else went ahead to Aaru Pokhari. Fortunately, we had materials in the medical bag for making a cast, so I could do that if necessary to get her on her feet again.

As the team prepared to leave, I chatted with Ann, who had made it clear that she was impatient, wanting to get back to Gorkha. "I feel like a filthy mess," she said, tightening her lips in a look of disgust, slowly shaking her head. "It's been over two weeks since I've showered. I don't know how you stand it."

I smiled sympathetically, realizing how long ago I had given up the idea of regular showers. While we were in the field, bathing was either at a local water tap, Nepali-style, or from a basin in the privacy of the tent.

As the team bustled off over the hill, I felt an unusual sense of peace settle over me. I was cheery at the prospect of having, just this once, an actually restful break from the relentless routine. I took a look at Sundaree's ankle, assessing the damage. It was still swollen, but there was no bruising, and I felt certain it wasn't broken.

Our camp was near a small settlement of Gurung families. Sundaree hobbled over to chat with an elderly grandmother who was sitting on their veranda grinding roasted corn, which would likely be used to make the local beer. A little girl playing nearby had a heavy layer of dust and dirt on every bit of skin that was visible. She wore a dress that looked like more dirt than fabric, and a favorite saying of my mother's came to mind: "Put those pants in the wash—they're so filthy they would stand alone!" I listened in on the conversation.

"*Aamaa, buccha-haaru, kina na dhune?*" Sundaree asked the woman, with a sweet, inquiring smile belying what was to me the rudeness of the question. *Why don't the children bathe?*

Her school-age grandson, standing nearby, piped up, "My mother says it gives us fever."

The grandmother laughed. "Yes, and I found out that it gave me diarrhea, so I stopped too," she answered. She was pleasant and seemed not at all offended by the discussion, happy to chat for the next half hour or so. I learned again that people have reasons for what they do, or don't do.

Late in the morning Ram and I went out foraging for firewood, and he cooked a lunch of fried rice from last night's leftovers. I was overjoyed to spend the afternoon around the cooking fire reading, finishing up paperwork, and writing letters. As the sun started to approach the tops of the mountains behind us, I moved into my tent for a nap before dinner. Even though I was barely able to stretch out under the sky-blue nylon dome, it was the ultimate luxury—a siesta. I lay back against the rolled-up sleeping bag. Sundaree and Ram chatted quietly in the distance, preparing the evening meal and discussing our return to Gorkha village. Birds screeched loudly nearby. The river below purred. Flies buzzed urgently, trying to find entry into my tent.

Suddenly, "Mary Anne Didi, *khanna tayarri bhayo!*" chirped Sundaree. *Food is ready!* I roused from my nap and emerged from the tent, ready for the familiar ritual of *dal bhat*.

Our cheerful mood continued through the evening's rice and dal. Though any vegetables were long since used up, we were so overjoyed at the leisurely day that it was unthinkable to complain about anything.

I asked Sundaree and Ram if they were anxious to get home from this long trip.

"Oh, yes, my little boy is wanting to see me, I think," Sundaree replied. Her sweet, heart-shaped face beamed as she mentioned her son. As was typical for many Nepali families, the lure of paid employment was often great enough that children, even small ones, were left at home in the care of other family members when the mothers went away to work.

"He's home with your husband?" I continued. I had met Sundaree's husband once, a much older man who had a reputation for being a *raaksi-kaani manche,* a drinking man. I felt a sudden tension in the air and realized that I had asked an inappropriate question. Sundaree nodded and smiled faintly, looking down at her food, and Ram quickly busied himself with bringing more rice.

"Bhat, Didi?" asked Ram. And the subject was closed.

Ram told me about his wedding planned for the following year, an arranged marriage but one he approved. I asked their thoughts about the new nurses, and both agreed that over time, they would get used to the work, it would all be okay. They asked about my plans for the next few months in Kathmandu. Exactly what I would be doing for the Foundation there was not clear, so I gave some vague answers and we finished eating in silence.

After retiring to my tent, I thought briefly about the evening's discussion. There must be problems with Sundaree's husband, I mused. When I was in Kathmandu several months later, Corinne came by after a visit to Gorkha with news of our field staff. It seemed that the husband was indeed an alcoholic and also had been abusive. During their first treks with us, Sundaree and Kiran, the newest porter, had fallen in love. Not long after I left Gorkha, they both had resigned from the work and moved in together. Corinne didn't know if Sundaree had been able to take her young son with her when she left; the decision would have been her husband's.

Wow. Friendships among the team were indeed many and shifting. But Sundaree was fairly new to the team, and I had never noticed anything unusual about her relationships with the others. But this was the classic story that could happen anywhere in the world: two people who worked together falling into a forbidden love. I'd suddenly zoomed far into the heavens and was looking back at the masses of humanity on every continent, and could see them all going through all the same changes: birth, love, anger, jealousy, pain, and death.

I was gripped with thoughts about Sundaree's dilemma for a

long time after hearing the story. Her decision to defy the dictates of custom, culture, family, and probably her own conscience if she had to leave her child was enormous. Her rights as a Nepali woman were very few. Her place in Nepali society was essentially as chattel of her husband, without access to property or decision-making apart from him. The courage it took, the angst she must have felt, was both distressing and inspiring. *Sweet Sundaree! Kasto dukkha,* I thought. *So much pain.* And also—*good for you, girl*!

But on that last trek, I knew nothing of the drama my young friend was living.

That night, for the first time in weeks, rather than falling asleep I began to think about the rest of the world, the life I might have outside the endless trails, these singular people. Before long I'd be launched back into where I'd come from. I had a brief flash of the San Francisco world from just a year ago: high-rise apartment buildings, pedigreed dogs sporting jeweled collars, traffic jams, and department stores packed with a dozen models of toasters. Would I ever fit into that world again? What did I want from the life that would come next? What could the "new me" do with what I had learned here?

Inevitably, thoughts about the looming future led me down the rocky path of remembering more of what I had left behind. My marriage was truly over, but as I ran my fingers along the silky tent skin, I was suddenly seized with the need to have a man in my life once more. Every inch of me ached to be held, to be enclosed in someone's muscular embrace. Would there ever be that someone again?

My future was, once more, as uncharted as the snowy peaks I could see through the open tent flap. Where would this experience, which so transformed my understanding of the world, be useful? I was ready to begin molding the life I wanted, not just yearning for the past I'd lost. I didn't understand then the immense importance that this time in Nepal would have for my future life, both who I would become and what I would do.

The following morning Sundaree's ankle swelling was diminished, and I was able to put a simple cast on it, with a walking heel that Ram carved out of a piece of firewood. By midafternoon we broke camp and started off to meet the rest of the team in Aru Pokhari. From there it would be an easy one-day trek back to Gorkha village and the comforts of the home I would soon be leaving.

Chapter 25
The Sari Rebellion

The porters stood before me in the equipment room at the office, quiet, solemn, ready for a face-off.

They had come to arrange supplies for the next day's final trek to Barpak, to be led this time by Jean and Ann. *Dokos*, duffle bags, cooking pots, bags of rice, and tent pieces were strewn about the room, ready to be packed up. I looked around with a surge of nostalgia: I would not be on this trip. It was the moment I'd longed for countless times, and here it was: My trekking days in Gorkha were over. This was the last time I'd see the team before I left for my new assignment in Kathmandu.

But something was brewing. Bhim Raj stepped forward and said he needed to speak with me.

"Mary Anne Didi," he started solemnly. "In our culture it is not proper for a Nepali man to carry a woman's clothing. We need to tell the Foundation that we cannot do that. It is important to us. We will need to quit this job if we have to carry saris." He stepped back to a deep silence, as the group awaited my response.

It seemed I had one more lesson to learn from my time here, and it had to come just as I was congratulating myself on a job well done.

Sita and the other staff hovered in the doorway. Sita had told me that to avoid conflict, the women on the team said they would carry their own saris. But she also noted they were sure that someone else was behind the scenes, twisting what was not a genuine cultural issue into a problem. Without using his name, it was clear they thought Captain Limbu was the mastermind of the porters' revolt. Captain was curiously not there that morning.

Since it had come up on the first Barpak trek, we'd never discussed the sari-carrying issue with the team, as several Nepali informants had assured us that porters' carrying saris in their *dokos* was not a cultural taboo. We had even asked other Gorkha-based porters, and none said it was a concern. I stood still for a moment, wrestling with a barrage of conflicting emotions. Sadness—*Bhim Raj, how could you? These are my guys! How can this come at the very end of my time with you?* Leaving would be hard enough, but now this?

I was angry as well. I suspected that Captain Limbu was trying to inflate his importance, this time by leading these good men into a dead-end showdown. Questionable behavior with the porters was a pattern we'd begun to see with Captain, but this time it was not just a minor matter.

I also felt a deep sympathy for these men, my friends. I fervently wished that they were asking for something I could help them fight for—more money, limits on the weight they had to carry. But not this made-up rebellion, which also blatantly pointed out the abysmally low status of women in this society. Women couldn't prepare food while they were menstruating, and in many households they had to reside separately in a small hut during that time. Anything related to women's reproductive functions, including menstruation, was considered "unclean" to Hindus, kept separate from men.

I knew I couldn't do what I wanted to do: meet the porters halfway, tell them we would find another solution, a compromise. In addition to hearing from my own Nepali sources that there was no cultural basis for their claim, I also had orders from our headquarters to hold firm. As porters, they needed to carry what they were asked to carry. And it was not a bluff—Gorkha had many porters who would be eager to take their places. As much as I would hate to choose strangers for the team, I knew that it could easily be done.

I felt a surge of adrenalin, powering my determination to manage this crisis respectfully, but firmly. I inhaled deeply and answered Bhim Raj.

"Bhim Raj, and everyone. I'm very sorry that you have this problem. But we have consulted many Nepalis who have told us that what you are saying is not true about your culture. If you believe it's true, then you must resign. We need porters who will carry whatever they need to carry."

Bhim Raj looked back at his troops. "Okay, Memsaab, then we can't come tomorrow," he said solemnly. I noticed that he had reverted to the old formal way of addressing me, distancing us: I was the Memsaab, of a superior status, rather than Didi. Okay, that was fair. There was a stir of mutterings from the porters who watched intently, some shaking their heads, some looking pained and confused.

Mek and Thul Bahadur, the most senior members of the team, looked around at the group, gave a quick "*Hunchha, bholi auchhu,*" —*Okay, I'll come tomorrow*—and moved out the door. The others continued to glance around at each other, looking distinctly uncomfortable.

"I understand. If you decide that you can't work tomorrow, then we will have a letter of resignation ready for you to sign," I said softly and with what I hoped was a sympathetic tone. "You can think it over, and we'll see you tomorrow morning at eight o'clock, as usual."

The group filed out quietly, and I looked around at the staff left in the room, shaking my head. I suddenly felt weak-kneed.

"You did well, Mary Anne Didi," said Sita. "I know they don't want to quit. But maybe some will. Captain should have been here today."

The other vaccinators nodded. Kaliwati, with grown children of her own, had her typical look of motherly annoyance, with a slight undertone of amusement. I could hear her thinking, *Those boys!*

The other nurses still hovered in the doorway. Jean was the first to ask for more background on the issue. "So, what was that really about?" she asked, sounding both bewildered and suspicious that she had missed something important. I could remember only too well the frustration of just partially understanding a conversation, getting most of the words but missing the main meaning.

I gave a quick summary of the conversation and the history behind "the sari issue," and dragged myself upstairs to my bedroom to escape.

Suddenly overwhelmed with exhaustion, I needed desperately to curl up and shut out the world. I sank onto my bed and closed my eyes, trying to relax the tension in every muscle, to calm my thoughts. But nothing could relieve me of the memory of Bhim Raj's face, his slightly desperate look of ambivalence and at the same time a determination—to do what? *To be a man*, I thought, in a society where so many men have little chance to do that, to be as good as the next man. Nepal was an unequal society in multiple ways—rich and poor, high caste and low caste, men and women. Porters were at the bottom of the male social ladder, with very little control over their lives. Of course they wanted that bit of empowerment that would come from taking a stand.

And who was I, a foreigner, a woman of privilege, to hand down a decision that would reduce their self-esteem? Social status often means self-respect, and a low position in society taints virtually every aspect of people's lives. Self-esteem and social pride helps all of us respond better to the endless challenges of life. And, no surprise, when men feel respected and valued, they don't have the same need to dominate or abuse women.

To quash the uneasy, queasy feeling in my stomach, I went for a long walk with Sita that afternoon. We talked about her plans, her family.

"I'll be staying with Corinne for a few weeks in Kathmandu," I told her. "Maybe you can come again to visit us?"

She gave a slight Nepali nod. "Maybe," she said. "It's so far from here." I understood that the distance she mentioned wasn't only geographic. In fact, many years would pass before we met again. We parted with a simple, "See you tomorrow."

The next morning, I heard the team gathering in the room below. After a quick breakfast, I pulled myself together, took three deep breaths to calm my nerves, and stepped into the equipment room. All nine of the expected porters seemed to be there. A surge of hope— *maybe they're all going!*

Then the two youngest men, charming Dil Man and baby-faced Bhakta, came forward and said, almost in unison, *"Jannu sakdaina."* *I can't go.*

Bhakta had a passive, polite demeanor, and I remembered that he had talked about going back to work with his father. But Dil Man's eyes were anguished. He glanced at me with what seemed a sense of betrayal, on whose part I wasn't sure, then quickly looked away.

I stood stone-faced, wanting to cry, while Ann held resignation forms out to the two young men. They each scratched a hurried "X" and went out the door into the sunny day, not looking back.

The remaining men stood silently for a moment, not meeting my eyes, then set about sorting equipment and organizing their *dokos*. The older porters, Bhim Raj among them, had reluctantly agreed to work, faced with the reality of families to support. One went out to recruit two substitutes for Bhakta and Dil Man.

There was no sense of celebration in the preparations that morning, none of the joking and fun that usually accompanied travel days. Leaving Ann in charge of final checks, I slunk back to my room to ponder what had just happened. Deep sighs. *Why do I feel so awful when I did the right thing, and in the end most of them decided to stay?* I wondered. Realizing that there had been no good choices, I also vowed that I'd do whatever was needed to avoid being in such a painful situation ever, ever again.

After some time, I heard shuffling noises indicating that the team was ready to leave, so I went down to the yard for a farewell. As they filed out of the gate I gave the Nepali "go well" to each small group, receiving some smiles and the occasional "Bye-bye" in return.

Sita gave me an extra long, extra deep namaste with her usual quizzical smile. *"Pheri betaulau, eh?"* she said softly. *See you again?*

As Bhim Raj walked by, he gave me a polite Nepali farewell with a sad smile, *"Raamro sanga bosnuhos,* Mary Anne Didi." *Stay well.*

"Raamro sanga jannuos, Bhim Raj Daai," I replied, the traditional goodbye when someone departs. *Go well.* Then they were gone.

Seeing these friends march down the path and out of my sight for the last time, I had a sharp jolt of reality. This was the hardest thing I'd done in my entire time in Nepal. I was losing not only the friendship of these warm and considerate people, but also my illusions that simply caring people-to-people would overcome the massive forces that separated us. Only genuine changes in who controlled our worlds would do that, and my efforts in Nepal were far removed from that process.

Several years later I had vivid memories of our porters' "sari rebellion" when a bloody, protracted Maoist insurgency was launched in Nepal, with some of its roots in Gorkha. Centuries of domination by the king or the Ranas, leaving the vast majority of the population desperately poor, finally became intolerable. Strikes by porters on various small expeditions were fairly common occurrences then too.

It was a period of general unrest in the country, of great hope for change, and the porters were the vanguard, showing us that it would happen. The ten-year war that ensued destabilized the monarchy, leading to its eventual overthrow. By the time peace accords were signed in 2006, thousands had died, and the Maoists claimed control of over 80 percent of the rural areas.

The revolution did bring some improvements—weakening of the caste system, a new constitution that gave more rights to women. But massive inequalities continue, as they do in most countries. Although I didn't think in those terms at the time, I was in fact simply part of a system that had for centuries perpetuated gross imbalances in power and privilege. The Nepali porters were poor and lacked power because other Nepalis were rich and powerful, and Nepal as a country was poor because other countries were rich and more powerful.

The inequities that I saw in Nepal—and that I was part of—have stayed with me in a visceral way. I've come to see that no important issue in global health or development is without a prominent element of inequality at its base. I was face to face with it that day in Gorkha.

During my remaining few days in the village, surprises continued. It had been a hot and dry June. The crops were in danger of failing, the corn especially, if the monsoon rains didn't come soon. I mentioned something about the weather to Gannu one day, and she told me in clear terms that the drought was because the gods were angry with people in Gorkha, who were too worldly.

"They drink *raksi*, they don't do their regular *pujahs*, they eat meat, and we don't know what else," she said vehemently. Shortly afterward I heard the familiar sounds of a local procession coming along the path by the house. A Nepali band was approaching, with horns blasting and a drum pounding, led by a wailing clarinet-like instrument. I raced out to the porch to see what was happening, Gannu joining me.

We watched the procession pass by the house. Behind a Brahmin priest chanting prayers marched a contingent of raucous, singing townspeople. On both sides of the road, neighbors stood holding buckets and, as the group approached, the entourage was splashed with water amid whoops of laughter. I looked at Gannu, puzzled. *Whaaat?*

"It's a rain ceremony, Memsaab," she said, with a look of supreme satisfaction. "They are going to the temple and will do a big *pujah* there."

Of course! The town was seeding the air for rain, trying to coax a miracle out of the forces that governed their world. I appreciated the logic of it and went back into the house for my weekly letter writing.

Less than thirty minutes later, I glanced out the window. Soft, fluffy white clouds had been replaced by giant, ominous black ones. Before long, the skies opened up with a massive, satisfying thunder-and-lightning storm. The monsoon had begun at last. Persistent leaks in the roof came back too—I quickly moved my bed to a safer corner of the room and set out buckets.

So there it was, prayers answered. The response of the rain gods had been so immediate, so definitive. Who could question it? And why would they, anyway? My Catholic upbringing had planted firmly in my consciousness the awareness that we can't necessarily see everything in the world that's real: the soul, the spirits of those who've left us. Why would the universe include only Christian mysteries?

When dawn brightened my room the next morning, it was suddenly my last day in Gorkha. I set out in the afternoon to say my goodbyes to the few townspeople I had gotten to know: Dr. K. C. and family, the mayor, some of the local shopkeepers. On my way back to the house I suddenly noticed a gaggle of kids following me who, as usual, were eager to practice their English.

"What-is-your-name?" was the usual question, with a staccato lift to each syllable. Then, "Where ees your home? What time ees eet?"

Any answer would bring peals of giggling and yet another question. When I looked at my watch and said, "Now it's twenty o'clock!" they howled with laughter, and eventually dropped back to pursue other games.

I knew I'd miss these kids. There were plenty of street children in Kathmandu, most begging for "one rupee." Those encounters were sad, when I thought about everything they lacked besides that rupee. But the kids in Gorkha hadn't learned that they were poor in relation to foreigners. They mostly knew that we had better English skills, something they all wanted, so our little interactions were lighthearted fun.

That evening after a final *dal bhat* dinner, I went to my room to pack for the next morning's trek back to the road. I could stow all my worldly possessions into a couple of duffle bags, and the collection looked pitifully small. After months of being bashed on the rocks for laundering and then dried in the sun, leached of most of their color, many of the few clothes I'd started with had become barely wearable. I'd learned to make do with so few accessories—a couple of ribbons to keep my hair out of my eyes, a solid water bottle, face cream, my dusty green REI daypack, the trusty Pentax camera, and a battered cassette player. My few souvenirs were all made in the villages: a small drum; a handmade wooden *teki* used for holding oil; some cotton cloth made in one of the villages. Half the weight seemed to be taken up with books, most for contribution to the shelves in the Kathmandu house.

Bags finally packed, I stepped out to the porch for one last look around at this place that had been home for the past year. After a hot day, the breeze was cool and sweet, the half-moon just rising over the dark hills. The guard chatted softly with a few passers-by who were heading home for the evening. I was filled with a vague sense of longing, trying to register that it was my last night here, that Gorkha would never again be home for me. I was leaving the team and the peace of the villages, taking with me what I had learned and the ways I'd changed in this one short year.

Only much later did I fully realize all that I'd gained from my time in Nepal. I'd spent a year in a world where spirits were as real as the trees, the birds, the rain. They affected life in every possible way: health, personal fortunes, interpersonal relationships, even the weather. Though I thought of them as mysterious superstitions when I first encountered them, I came to see that they were a familiar, comforting presence for people who wanted only to make sense of their daily reality. Any efforts to help people improve their lives, including their health, had to take into account the very different ways that people see the world. It was my most important lesson from that time.

But now, I was heading back to the noisy, dirty, sometimes exciting world of Kathmandu. Before long I'd go back to the West, which it seemed I'd left at least a century ago. I would not be the same person when I returned.

Epilogue

Nepal will always be my touchstone for understanding the wider world.

Those months in the villages of Gorkha district, immersed in the daily life of its people—their beauty and their pain—set the stage for what came next: my personal hopes, my career, and a vision of a life I could aim for. I wanted to continue to work toward improving the health of mothers and their children in other parts of the world. I wanted to support women like Maya and Maili to complete their pregnancies without the risk of bleeding to death or enduring days of labor with no one to assist. I wanted them to see their newborns live through those first critical days of life, able to grow older as happy kids. It turned out there was a name for that: *maternal and child health*.

Those hopes led me to graduate degrees and a career in international and global public health, with travel to many countries from a university base. I've been privileged to share what I've learned with hundreds of students over years of teaching. Even now, when I talk about the critical importance of health care for mothers and children, the images that come to me are often the Nepali women who had no recourse when their children were sick or their pregnancies went wrong. I'd seen firsthand how important women are for the health of families. Compounding their burdens, they often suffer from secondary status in societies dominated by men. Telling their stories became my most effective way to give students and others a tiny glimpse of that world.

Seeing the daily realities of Nepali hill people gave me a new appreciation for the concept of health as a basic right, not something only for people who can buy it. To make that "right" a reality requires services that reach those who need them the most. Information, medicines, support for health workers, and hospital care when needed shouldn't be a luxury. I grew to see that for any country, including my own, the right to health and health care is a vital aspect of human rights.

Nepal has stayed in my life in many other ways since my time in Gorkha. During my first week of graduate school at Johns Hopkins, I became close friends with a fellow Nepali student. Devi, his wife Munnu, and their three children became my surrogate family through most of my years in Baltimore, and enabled me to maintain a modicum of my Nepali language skills. I visited them several times after their return to Kathmandu.

In 2016, a year after the massive earthquake that had decimated much of the district, they went with me back to Gorkha. My aim was to find Sita, dear friend and team member, whom I'd not seen since leaving there. In the center of Gorkha village, we asked a small group of older women, seated on a low stone wall chatting together, if they knew her.

The response was immediate: "Yes, we can take you to her house!" One excited woman jumped into the car and directed us along the old path through town, the one I'd walked along so often, to a small storefront with living quarters in the back. We found a family member who went to fetch Sita from her garden plot nearby.

Twenty minutes later, I looked up to see an older woman with a bright red *tika* smudged on her forehead walking slowly up the path toward me. As she drew closer, I recognized those searching eyes and that quizzical smile. It was Sita.

"Mary Anne Didi, *ali moto bhayo*," she said with a sly smile. *You've gained a little weight.*

And just like that, we were together again, as if nearly forty years hadn't elapsed since we had last seen each other.

"And how good you look, Sita," I laughed, in my halting Nepali. We sank onto a bench, gazing at each other intently, as if trying to find that person we knew decades ago. "You remember me! How are you? It's been so many years!"

"Many years," she said. "I didn't think we would ever meet again."

Finding Sita, speaking with her after such a long time, had an edge of unreality at first. But when she came with me to the small hotel where we were spending the night, and we began sharing memories of the days when we had trekked and lived together, the elapsed years dropped away. Sita was living with extended family on her own property very near her parents' ancestral home. She had a large garden plot and a water buffalo that she milked faithfully twice daily.

As we spoke, with Sita once again filling in missing words of my halting sentences, I marveled at how successfully she had navigated life as a Nepali woman on her own terms. She had never married, instead choosing a career and economic independence. But she'd done it without sacrificing her family ties, her love of her home village, or even the agricultural traditions she'd grown up with. Sita's story gave me hope for the millions of other women who would need to slip off the constraints of their traditional cultures as they entered the modern age.

My time in Nepal also led to finding my lifetime partner, a man whose love for the country paralleled my own. With his knowledge of all things Nepali, which far surpasses mine, Stephen had published the first guide to trekking in Nepal. The name of our beautiful daughter echoes the endearment used for many little girls we met there: *Maia, love.* When Maia was six years old, we embarked on a family trek to the Everest region. Returning to that area, accompanied by my family, was an unsurpassed joy. I was once again truly on top of the world.

Acknowledgments

This story of my year in the villages of Nepal would never had taken shape without the guidance, support, and editing prowess of the talented women in my writing group. Brenda Peterson, who leads us, has inspired, encouraged, and informed my efforts to share that life-altering experience. Laura Foreman, Lindsay Pyfer, Margie Combs, Amanda Mander, and Marlene Blessing have been with me since the first words were set down and have offered invaluable editing assistance as well as moral support.

I had the good fortune to work with She Writes Press in the production of this book, supported by Publisher Brook Warner and Associate Publisher Lauren Wise. This hybrid press expertly guides women writers—both aspiring and already well-published—to share their stories, backed by an experienced editorial and production team. I am immensely grateful for their counsel and mentoring. I was also fortunate to have the expert assistance of Mary Bisbee-Beek in promoting my story.

During my time in Gorkha, my teammates, including Corinne Collins, Kate Jewell, and several short-term volunteers, were soul-saving sources of support as I worked my way through the year of discovery, exhaustion, and joy. The district physician Dr. K. C. helped me see what I could accomplish without advanced knowledge of tropical medicine. Getting to know my Nepali team of vaccinators,

porters, and advance men opened my eyes to many of the mysteries of the Nepali culture. In particular, Sita Devi Khadka was a valued sister and friend.

I was fortunate to volunteer with Dooley Foundation, now Dooley-Intermed, for my work in Nepal. Stella Saint was the Foundation's understanding and empathetic country director. The late Dr. Verne Chaney was especially foresightful in encouraging me to further my education, which led to public health degrees and eventually a university career.

My dear friends Dr. Devi and Munnu Shrestha and their children have fostered my continued connection with Nepal since I met them in graduate school. They have kept me in their family and in touch with Nepal over the years.

It is to my own family that I owe the deepest gratitude. My dear late parents supported my desire to venture away from rural Montana and experience the larger world. My daughter, Maia, and stepson, Michael, are enduring reminders of the joys of family. My husband, Stephen Bezruchka, is my unfailing resource for all things Nepali, and I am immensely grateful for his steadfast encouragement, love, and support.

About the Author

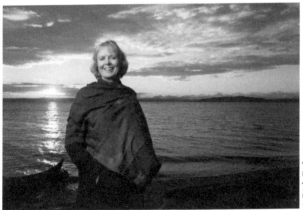

© Rick Dahms

Mary Anne Mercer grew up on a Montana ranch and has spent most of her career working in public health in countries around the globe. A writer and activist, she coedited *Sickness and Wealth: The Corporate Assault on Global Health* and has published extensively in the *Huffington Post* on issues of social justice and health. Excerpts from her book have appeared in *Tikkun* magazine, the *Communion Arts Journal*, and in the book *Secret Histories: Stories of Courage, Risk, and Revelation*. She received a 2012 Silver Solas Award from Travelers' Tales for "Best Travel Writing" and the 2015 inaugural award for "Communicating Public Health to the Public" from the University of Washington.

SELECTED TITLES FROM SHE WRITES PRESS

She Writes Press is an independent publishing company founded to serve women writers everywhere. Visit us at www.shewritespress.com.

Naked Mountain: A Memoir by Marcia Mabee $16.95, 978-1-63152-097-6
A compelling memoir of one woman's journey of natural world discovery, tragedy, and the enduring bonds of marriage, set against the backdrop of a stunning mountaintop in rural Virginia.

Gap Year Girl by Marianne Bohr $16.95, 978-1-63152-820-0
Thirty-plus years after first backpacking through Europe, Marianne Bohr and her husband leave their lives behind and take off on a yearlong quest for adventure.

Peanut Butter and Naan: Stories of an American Mother in The Far East by Jennifer Magnuson $16.95, 978-1-63152-911-5
The hilarious tale of what happened when Jennifer Magnuson moved her family of seven from Nashville to India in an effort to shake things up—and got more than she bargained for.

The Coconut Latitudes: Secrets, Storms, and Survival in the Caribbean by Rita Gardner $16.95, 978-1-63152-901-6
A haunting, lyrical memoir about a dysfunctional family's experiences in a reality far from the envisioned Eden—and the terrible cost of keeping secrets.

This is Mexico: Tales of Culture and Other Complications by Carol M. Merchasin $16.95, 978-1-63152-962-7
Merchasin chronicles her attempts to understand Mexico, her adopted country, through improbable situations and small moments that keep the reader moving between laughter and tears.

This Trip Will Change Your Life: A Shaman's Story of Spirit Evolution by Jennifer B. Monahan $16.95, 978-1-63152-111-9
One woman's inspirational story of finding her life purpose and the messages and training she received from the spirit world as she became a shamanic healer.